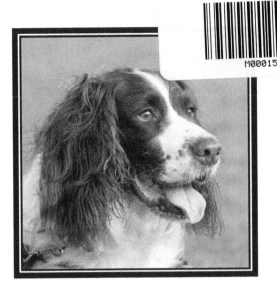

The HAPPY English Springer Spaniel

Raise a Happy, Well-Mannered Dog and Avoid
Dog Behavior Professionals for Life

- 🐾 Dog Happiness Tips
- 🐾 Techniques for a Well-behaved English Springer Spaniel
- 🐾 Prevent Behavior Issues
- 🐾 Fulfill Your Puppy's Needs
- 🐾 Be the Ideal Guardian
- 🐾 Avoid Common Mistakes

Asia Moore

Dog Behavior Expert & Acclaimed Author

*"Dogs are small rays of light caught on the Earth
a short time to brighten our days."*
— Unknown

Preface

It takes time, commitment, tenacity, consistency and knowledge to raise a happy and healthy English Springer Spaniel that doesn't suffer from health and behavioral issues.

This book is NOT like most other breed-specific books, because we believe that it's far better for all parties concerned (human and canine) to **prevent** problems rather than suffering the frustrations of living with or learning how to eliminate problems and rehabilitate an English Springer Spaniel that has already developed health or behavioral issues.

It is always better to prevent unwanted behaviors than to hope you, or someone else, may have what it takes to eliminate them in the future, after your family is at their wits end, your neighbors hate you, your friends no longer visit, your dog has been deemed aggressive or dangerous, and you're having guilty thoughts of re-homing every time you drive past your local SPCA.

 If you want a happy, well-mannered canine companion to be a loyal, well-behaved and valued member of your

family, it absolutely DOES matter how you raise your dog.

Every breed has uniquely different talents and needs. Even those that were once primarily working dogs that have become companion breeds.

As an example, the Border Collie is a very smart, high-energy working dog that excels at the job of herding. Therefore, if you expect this dog to sit around doing nothing all day while you're at work, you will most likely return to holes in your drywall, torn apart couches and a home that looks like it's been through a cyclone.

On the other hand, the Shih Tzu lap dog, which was originally only permitted to be owned by royalty, sat on silk pillows, and was used to warm beds, has vastly different daily exercise requirements, and would be a poor choice for someone requiring a companion that could protect them from being mugged on streets ravaged by gang warfare.

The eager to please English Springer Spaniel was originally a flushing and retrieving gun dog, that is now a furry companion for many humans.

This dog is literally capable of learning anything you have the time, inclination and skill level to teach and the more the better, as this canine loves to please, and is always eager for a new challenge.

Friendly, sociable and people-oriented, this dog requires a moderate to high amount of daily exercise so that they do not become bored and overweight. In order to raise a happy and healthy fur friend, you need to be totally honest with yourself and absolutely certain that you have the lifestyle and energy needed for properly caring for this energetic canine companion.

If you're looking for a playful and active canine companion with a loving and endearing personality to share your life with, whether you're into canine sports or hiking your local trails, this amiable, eager to learn and willing to please dog that loves spending time with their family may be perfect for you.

While still admired for their flushing and retrieving abilities, once socialized and trained, this spaniel will be a loyal, friendly and obedient family companion that is always eager to do whatever is asked of them.

Usually gentle with children and when properly trained and socialized will also get along easily with other dogs and pets. This dog is a steady and dependable field dog as well as a wonderful family companion for both the young and young at heart.

Versatile and successful in many different roles, this loving dog has tireless enthusiasm and may be the perfect companion for a family with someone who works at home, is retired, or may even be a first-time canine guardian, so long as they are consistently firm with rules and boundaries.

FACT *This dog will almost certainly become overweight if they do not receive adequate daily exercise. Most English Springer Spaniels are sturdy, yet gentle dogs that are great for children old enough to respect a dog's space. This dog will be a faithful and loving companion always eager for the next adventure.*

Every dog breed has different talents and needs and when you decide to share your life with a particular breed, if you want a happy and well-adjusted companion, you must also be prepared to provide your dog with what he or she needs to be a happy member of your family.

FACT *Almost all canine problems, both mentally and physically, are a direct result of lack of knowledge or unwillingness on the part of the human guardian to choose the right dog for their particular energy and lifestyle. It takes research, time and commitment to learn what each dog truly needs.*

This book is uniquely different, and humans reading it need to clearly understand that the pages of this book are not all about describing what to do to eliminate problematic canine behaviors that have already occurred.

Rather, the main focus of this breed-specific book is to describe what the human guardian needs to understand and commit to doing on a daily basis in order to match the English Springer Spaniel's needs, so that they can raise a happy, healthy and well-behaved dog that never has to experience behavioral issues.

FACT *While still registered together, for the past 70 years the English Springer breed has been separated into show lines and working or field lines that are quite different from one another, to the point of the gene pools being almost totally separate from one another.*

Do not expect this book to be like all the others that set out endless correlations between specific mal-behaviors and what steps or actions the human guardian can take in an attempt to correct them.

In other words, this book is a totally new slant on raising a happy and healthy English Springer Spaniel, because the main focus here is on the prevention of behavioral issues rather than addressing them after they have already surfaced.

About the Author

Asia Moore

Dog Behavior Expert & Acclaimed Author

Ever since my first birthday, I was immersed in nature, and have always enjoyed a special connection with all creatures, both great and small. I learned to communicate and "talk" with many animals in their language, both wild and domesticated. At approximately the age of twelve, dogs began to become the main focus of my life, when I set about training and grooming my first puppy.

When friends and neighbors began to recognize how well behaved my dog was, and were subsequently impressed with all the tricks and routines she could perform, often without a spoken word, they asked me to train their dogs, too.

I count myself very fortunate to have experienced the unconditional love of so many dogs over the years, all of who taught me many different life lessons. I began this journey with my first mixed breed ("Cindy") who protected me from my marauding brothers, then my mixed breed ("Pepper") who had an amazing human vocabulary and always knew when someone was not to be trusted, my Blue Heeler ("Bugsy") who would hike endless trails and swim miles with me, to my current loving Shih Tzu ("Boris") and all my clients' dogs in between.

Now, some 40 years later, and endless different breeds, including these patient and affectionate clowns of the dog world, and many hybrids and mutts, from tiny Chihuahuas to bouncing Belgians, a cascade of fur friends have passed through my life.

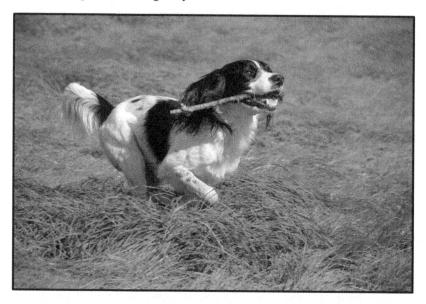

For the last 40 years, I have been managing my dog whispering, dog sitting and matchmaking businesses and have enjoyed countless experiences working with dogs of all breeds and their guardians. While life may sometimes bring us struggles and setbacks, I've never stopped learning from the many dogs that have graced my life, and I've always loved and been passionate about what I do.

All these years of experience taught me invaluable lessons in all aspects of the human-canine relationship interaction. For instance, I learned how to effectively communicate with our canine friends, understand their needs and help them and their guardians lead a fulfilling and happy life together. *What could be better than that?*

While clients' dogs now remain the focal point of my dog whispering, sitting and grooming life, I also focus on writing books where my goal is to pass on my knowledge and experience to all responsible dog owners (**Must Have Publishing.com**). At the same time, I continue to train human guardians, so that they can improve their relationships with their dogs and understand how to prevent and alleviate behavioral issues (**K-9 Super Heroes Dog Whispering.com**), and how to easily find excellent products their dog needs (**AskBoris.com**).

Also, I have an online matchmaking service (**Knows To Nose.com**) to help humans "know" how to choose the right dog "nose" for their energy and lifestyle, before they make the wrong decision and end up with troubling problems.

I am also often called upon to speak to groups about the changing roles for the canine population and how they now fit into our modern world. As well, I help humans and their chosen canines establish harmonious relationships with neighbors for those residing in multi-family living situations, such as apartment and condominium complexes.

I feel blessed that the canine world has been a major part of my life for so many years, as it never gets old, and it's always an opportunity to learn something new. I continuously stay in touch with my clients through my business websites and personal consultations and I love how every unique dog/human relationship brings new lessons to light and enhances everyone's life in untold, indescribable ways.

*I'd like to thank you for purchasing "**The Happy English Springer Spaniel**" and reassure you that the pages of this book contain the distilled knowledge of over 40 years experience, which, by the way, includes helping a nervous dog suffering from anxiety about crossing over unfamiliar, slippery floor tiles.*

When taken to heart, the knowledge, tips and techniques in this book can help you along your special journey inside the amazing world of our canine friends, so that you can know the unconditional love, special bond and joy that only our four-legged companions selflessly offer to us flawed humans.

Visit Asia online at the following .com locations:

www.K-9SuperHeroesDogWhispering.com
www.KnowsToNose.com
www.MustHavePublishing.com
www.AskBoris.com

Table of Contents

Chapter 1: Introduction

"Properly trained, a man
can be dog's best friend."
— Corey Ford

The purpose of this book is to focus on the important steps the humans in this relationship really need to be aware of and commit to providing in order to ensure that this smallest of the herding dogs can live a happy and healthy life, which in turn will ensure a happy relationship for everyone.

Even though humans and dogs have been relying on one another for more than 30,000 years, it's still highly important that you take an honest look at your life, decide whether sharing your life with a dog is truly feasible, and then if it is, choose the companion that is best suited to your particular lifestyle.

Within the pages of this book you will find information to help you choose wisely by providing you with a clear understanding concerning whether or not YOU have what it takes to be the right match for raising a happy and well-mannered English Springer Spaniel companion.

In addition, this book describes in detail what the human guardian needs to keep in mind and commit to doing on a daily basis in order to match this friendly and loving companion's needs, so that they can raise a happy, healthy and well-behaved dog that never has to experience behavioral issues.

All the information, suggestions, tips and advice given in this publication is the result of more than 40 years' experience helping humans positively and effectively interact with the canine world.

If you take all that is written on these pages to heart, and regularly and consistently apply them, your active, fun-loving and loyal English Springer Spaniel will be a happy family member that will not have to suffer from any behavioral problems. In other words, the focus is placed on prevention, rather than trying to correct any issues after they have surfaced.

Every Chapter of this book contains valuable information that will provide you with a solid understanding of the breed and the steps you need to take to raise a happy and well-behaved companion.

For instance, **Chapter 2** – *"Asia's Happiness Tips"* sets out a summary of what she personally believes makes for a happy English Springer

Spaniel and encourages you to ask yourself what YOU think would make this dog happy.

Chapter 3 – *"Overview of the Happy English Springer Spaniel"* will outline vital statistics, coat colors and common features, intelligence, temperament and interesting secrets and facts that may not be commonly known. Further, in order to raise a contented dog, you need to have some basic knowledge of the interesting history of the English Springer Spaniel breed, to help you choose wisely so that you are able to better comprehend this dog's needs.

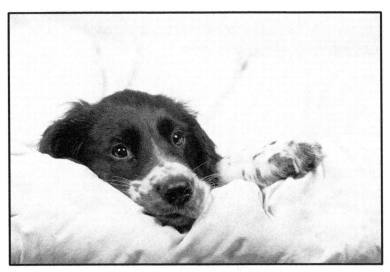

Chapter 4 – *"Healthy English Springer Spaniel = Happy Dog"* is where you will find out what you need to know about medical care, safety and health issues that may affect this medium-sized breed, including common diseases and viruses, allergies and canine CPR procedures that could save a life. Needless to say, if your dog is not physically healthy, he or she will not be a happy canine companion for very long, because suffering from health-related issues will undoubtedly create a miserable and ill-mannered dog.

In **Chapter 5** – *"Let Your Dog BE a Happy Dog"*, you will find information about how to let your English Springer Spaniel actually BE a dog, rather than attempting to turn them into a fur human, which can make for a very confused, unhappy and ill-mannered canine.

Chapter 6 – *"Every Happy English Springer Spaniel Wants Exercise"*, first outlines some of the original history of this dog when they were originally Standard sized working dogs, so that while still being an energetic dog that loves to run and play, has become more of a companion; if you know what they were bred to do, you will better understand how important it is to commit to the daily exercise routines recommended in this book, without which the English Springer Spaniel will not be happy or healthy for very long.

Chapter 7 – *"Feeding the Happy English Springer Spaniel"*, is where you will find information about the structure of the canine jaw, various food options and feeding suggestions as well as treats to avoid for raising a happy and healthy companion.

In **Chapter 8** – *"Care of the Happy English Springer Spaniel"*, you will find travel safety tips, licensing, insurance, essential grooming procedures and important care of nails, ears, teeth and paws, all of which will help you to raise a happy and healthy dog.

While some of this information might seem generic, imagine how you might feel going for months without washing your hair, cutting your nails or brushing your teeth. Unfortunately, that is the reality for many dogs, because their owners have not been properly advised with respect to the importance of good grooming habits. How happy and well behaved do you think such a poorly cared for English Springer Spaniel would be?

Chapter 9 – *"Are YOU the Ideal Happy English Springer Spaniel Guardian?"* is concerned with asking yourself some serious questions, including whether your energy, activity, commitment and lifestyle matches what this dog needs to be happy and well behaved. It's vital for you to give serious consideration to these questions when considering any breed, because should you choose the wrong dog to share your life with, everybody will be miserable.

Chapter 10 – *"Humans Make a LOT of Stupid Mistakes"* outlines that far too often we humans, without even realizing it, are the cause of creating behavioral problems in our canine companions. You will find out what are some of the common mistakes to avoid (and the right thing to do!) when it comes to socialization, accidental rewards, fear of noises, the right collars, basic rules and boundaries, adolescent craziness and more.

 Simply being aware of the many mistakes we humans can often inadvertently be guilty of when raising our canine companions, can mean the difference between a Happy English Springer Spaniel with no behavioral issues or a life of frustration and correction.

Chapter 11 – *"Happy English Springer Spaniel Body Language"*, outlines the basics of learning canine body language, and will help you be safe around other dogs. Learning to properly "read" a dog's intentions can prevent an unwanted encounter with another canine or human, and this will help to ensure that everyone remains safe and happy.

In Chapter 12 – *"Training Basics for a Happy English Springer Spaniel",* you will learn valuable training tips and routines that will help to keep your dog truly happy and well behaved for their entire life. It's no surprise that a properly trained dog will be a much happier companion that everyone enjoys being around, and will be far less likely to develop behaviour issues later in life.

Developing a basic training program and learning to teach your dog commands and discipline is all part of starting your dog off on the right paw.

Chapter 13 – *"What If You Slip Up?"* is only necessary because we humans tend to get too busy and overwhelmed with the rigors of daily living, which means we sometimes forget to be consistent with providing what our particular dog may need to be happy. If you slip up, this Chapter has outlined a few of the more common behavioral issues and how to quickly get yourself back on track.

Chapter 14 – *"Surprise Bonus Chapter"* is a Question and Answer section containing a few human/canine situations, with humans asking questions and wise words from the perspective of the dog, which answers the questions. You will also find an amusing and educational true story about a happy dog that just refused to set one paw on the newly installed tiles in his family home.

Take heed humans, because when you honestly assess your own compatibility, lifestyle and energy level for being the right guardian for the faithful English Springer Spaniel, and are vigilant about following the advice and tips outlined in the following pages, you can raise a healthy and happy dog that will be a joy to live with and will never have to suffer from any behavioral issues.

Chapter 2: Asia's Happiness Tips

*"Dogs do speak, but only to
those who know how to listen."*
— Orhan Pamuk

The following few paragraphs are a summary of my own personal ramblings, beliefs, and ideas about what I think makes for a happy English Springer Spaniel.

While I hope you may wholeheartedly agree, it's absolutely okay if you have other ideas, or if you may have an entirely different take on this subject, because we will all have our own "personal" ideas about what constitutes happiness for a smart and playful English Springer, and if your ideas are different from mine, this does not mean that they are any less valid.

If you're considering sharing your life with this intelligent canine and have never before really sat down and consciously thought about what would make this particular breed truly happy, while you may gain a little insight from reading about my own personal beliefs, I encourage you to take the time to do this exercise yourself. If you have a family, get them involved in this fun exercise, too.

When you take the time to sit with a piece of paper and pen and begin to write down what YOU think makes a Springer Spaniel happy, you may be surprised about what surfaces, and this simple exercise may inspire you and your family to discover new ways to bond with your dog, which will be the basis of having a truly happy relationship.

I'll help to get you started with the following question:
"What do you think would make an English Springer Spaniel happy?"

I've shared the last 14 years of my life with a wonderfully loving and well behaved Shih Tzu and I believe that the very best start you can make, with respect to "happiness" when first bringing home your new puppy is to do all you can to reassure him or her that they are not alone (see below).

Happy New Surroundings

The puppy will be understandably nervous about the new and unfamiliar faces, surroundings and smells, and will be missing their mother, other siblings and everything in their environment they had grown used to during their first 8 to 10 weeks of life.

Make sure that you don't overwhelm your new puppy with too much all at once. For instance, close off rooms that you don't need access to and encourage your puppy to come to you as you wander about in a smaller space.

Happy Sleep Patterns

When it's time to go to bed, take your puppy outside for a bathroom break, and then make sure that you have a nice, cozy kennel all ready for your new puppy with a soft lining or blanket and place their new kennel inside your bedroom, so that they will be able to hear and see you.

TIP *Unless you want your English Springer Spaniel to sleep on your bed when they're fully grown, even when they may have wet or dirty feet, or just rolled in a dead rat, now is the time to exercise a little tough love as the new puppy will most likely not want to be alone in their kennel and will prefer sleeping next to you.*

If your bed is large enough to accommodate their kennel, this is the best way to help your puppy have a happy sleep time because they will be next to you, but still safe inside their own kennel, and as they grow larger they will be used to their kennel and will not mind that it is sitting on the floor. Congratulations! You've just created a routine that will ensure happy and respectful sleeping patterns for your dog.

Happy Puppy Play

Taking the time for regular play sessions with your new Springer Spaniel puppy will certainly make them very happy, so make sure you set aside several times during your day when you stop with the human work and chores and engage your puppy in fun games for 5 or 10 minutes at least three or four times a day.

FACT *Every puppy and dog needs some time in their day where they can relax and play a fun game, and this is the beginning of trust and respect between you and your fur friend.*

Happy Puppy Housetraining

One of the very first things your new puppy needs to learn is where the bathroom is, and the more vigilant you are, the fewer "accidents" will occur, which will make both of you much happier.

I taught my Shih Tzu (Boris) to ring a little bell whenever he needed to go outside, which is a very valuable "trick" to teach. Just hang a loud ringing bell at the end of a ribbon, string or rope from the doorknob where you will always take your dog through to go outside for a bathroom break. Every time you take them out, go to the bell, lift their paw and knock it against the bell to make it ring. Say *"Good boy, or girl – go pee?"* Then immediately take them out through this door.

Learn to pay attention and understand your dog's body language, so that you can help teach them proper bathroom habits at a very young age. This is a very smart, eager to please dog and it should not be difficult to quickly train them that outside is where they need to go to get to their bathroom.

When they wake up in the morning, take them outside immediately. Twenty minutes after they have eaten a meal, take them outside to relieve themselves. After a play session or when they've had a big drink of water, or woken up from a nap, take them outside. After they've gone pee or number 2, immediately praise and reward them with a treat.

Yes, to do this right, you and your puppy will be spending a lot of time going outside, but once their bladder grows larger and stronger, the number of hours he or she can "hold" it will increase, and the number of times your dog will have to visit the great outdoor bathroom during each day will markedly decrease.

Use this bathroom training time also as a way to create a strong bond between you and your dog and as their first lessons in leash training and reward training for doing what you ask.

TIP *If you take the time to go out with them while they're on leash, it's easy to train your dog to "go" on command, and as they mature, you'll be very glad that you took the time to do this, especially if you live where there may be cold or wet winters.*

Happy Puppy Feeding

It's not rocket science to understand that providing your puppy or dog with the best nutrition from the very first day you bring them home will lead to a healthier fur friend, which in turn, will lead to a feel-good, energetic and happy companion.

Be aware of the importance of what you feed your dog and commit to doing the best you can to keep your canine friend healthy and happy. Read labels and feed them only the highest-quality food, so they have the best opportunity for a long life.

While it's important to start your puppy off with the right food, it's just as important to continue to feed your adult dog the very best diet. Please refer to Chapter 7 (Feeding the Happy English Springer Spaniel), where you will read about types of food, appropriate treats and more.

Happy Socializing

Socializing a new puppy is one of the most important steps you can take to ensure that your chosen companion lives a happy and stress-free life.

When you don't take the time to properly socialize your puppy, and indeed, keep on socializing throughout their lifetime, you can actually create many behavioral issues; some of these can be so severe that your dog may be in danger of having their life prematurely shortened. A normally gentle and loving dog, without proper rules and boundaries, this intelligent dog may quickly take over.

Many times, I've been called upon to help a human alleviate aggressive tendencies being displayed by their canine companion, and in pretty much every instance, this could have been entirely avoided if the dog had been properly trained and socialized.

In the case of the English Springer Spaniel, if you make the mistake of coddling and babying this companion and allowing him or her to be in control, you can end up creating a bossy dog that is downright disagreeable, with a reputation for being an *"armpit alligator"* (when they're still small enough to carry around) should anyone get too close.

Every dog must have a human leader to keep them safe and teach them appropriate rules and boundaries, and most dogs also require a significant amount of socializing, and more daily exercise and mental stimulation than you might imagine.

 This is a strong and active dog that will appreciate an energetic, activity-filled lifestyle.

The English Springer Spaniel will need to be well and continually socialized at a young age, and taught to keep their boundless enthusiasm under control. They will be interested participants that enjoy being involved in all of the family's activities, especially if they involve hiking, running, swimming, learning tricks, a canine sport, or plenty of varied outdoor adventures.

When not properly socialized, trained and taught to respect the word of their human guardians, this friendly companion has the smarts to become a bossy leader if their owner is not confident enough to be the leader that this dog can respectfully follow.

Without a human to trust, respect and follow, any dog can get themselves and their humans into all sorts of unwanted troubles. Often, dogs that do not have a human to lead them, even generally friendly ones like the English Springer Spaniel, can feel forced into acting out in an aggressive manner when they feel overly timid, shy, nervous or threatened.

Any sort of aggression is a huge stress on both dog and human and, as we are all aware, stress shortens lives and prevents anyone from

experiencing happiness, so help make your dog happy and make sure that you don't place the very heavy burden of making human decisions on the shoulders of your canine companion.

While early socialization of a puppy is very important, keep in mind that it's just as important to continue your adult dog's socialization throughout their lifetime. Please refer to Chapter 10 (Humans Make a LOT of Stupid Mistakes) that outlines the many aspects of socializing your English Springer Spaniel.

Happy Training

Almost as important as proper socializing to keep your dog happy, is proper training, which should never be overlooked, unless you want to create an unstable spaniel that ignores their humans, barks and growls at everything and thinks they are the boss of all they survey.

Eager to please, the hardworking, playful and obedient English Springer approaches life with a great sense of fun and adventure, and will usually be friendly toward other dogs (unless they have not been socialized). This is a dog that has a tireless enthusiasm and zest for life. A calm, structured living situation and a regular exercise routine will prevent anxiety and other behavioral problems that may stem from being under-challenged.

Although this is not a dog that must be strenuously exercised to the point of exhaustion every day, their original hunting bloodline does give them great stamina, which means that in order to maintain their health, regular daily exercise will prevent their tendency to become overweight. If allowed to become lazy and inactive, the English Springer will quickly gain weight, which can lead to problem health issues.

FACT *This spaniel is the oldest of all sporting gun dogs and is still admired for their outstanding ability to flush and retrieve downed game, as well as being a loyal, friendly and obedient family companion always eager to do what is asked of them.*

Depending on how curious they may be, how much exercise they normally receive outside of the home, and how strong their hunting desire, when not properly trained, this dog may ignore calls to come back when they are on the scent of something interesting.

Start training this companion as soon as you bring him or her home from the breeder and you will have given yourself the best opportunity to have a happy, eager to comply and safe companion at your side before they are six months old. Of course, you will start out with short training sessions of no more than 5 to 10 minutes at a time, and as they slowly mature, you can increase the length of your sessions.

Make sure any training is a fun and happy time for both you and your dog, with lots of happy praise and treats, and he or she will quickly learn to trust and respect you as their leader and be eager for their next session. This canine Einstein will be an easy to train dog that should catch on very quickly. Even young children can get in on the act and have fun teaching their loving fur friend basic tricks, such as shake a paw, sit, or roll over.

While this smart puppy can begin training at an early age, when you continue their training throughout their life, this enthusiastic and affectionate companion will usually be an eager participant that is entirely capable of learning endless commands, tricks, routines, and hand signals, as well as many canine sports. See more in Chapter 12 (Training Basics for a Happy English Springer Spaniel).

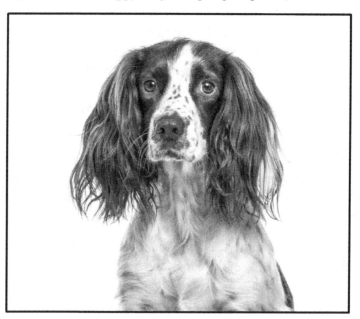

Happy Exercising

While the English Springer Spaniel is intelligent and versatile, which makes them successful in any different roles, and they enjoy learning new routines, they also need some down time, or some time off from your vigilant supervision.

 Just like us humans, who need time where they don't have to think about work, our dogs also need some free time where they can enjoy romping and playing with the family or exploring the local woodland paths, rolling in the grass or lazing in the warm sunshine, and just being a dog.

The English Springer Spaniel can be a moderate or highly energetic dog depending on their age. He or she will generally have a lively and playful temperament that loves to chase and romp, and depending on what you're into, the English Springer Spaniel may be a great hunting companion or a blue-ribbon performer in many different canine sports.

Supervision during play with other dogs is always important and in order to prevent possible squabbles, you will need to ensure that you intervene should your puppy or young dog try to be overly bossy with other dogs or is feeling overwhelmed by bigger dogs.

While every dog is different, with respect to how much exercise they might need, how active <u>YOU</u> are will also have a definite effect. You can learn much more about the exercises that will keep this dog happy in Chapter 6 (Every Happy English Springer Spaniel Wants Exercise).

Happy Visits to the Vet

Even though you may be feeding the best food, properly exercising, socializing and training your dog to be a calm and obedient member of your family, you will also want to have at least yearly visits to your chosen veterinarian's office to make sure all is well.

Start taking your dog to the vet's office even when they don't have any reason to be there, other than to receive a treat and friendly greetings, so that they get used to the different smells and people who work there because when you do this, your dog will learn that visits to the vet's office can be a happy time.

While it's ideal to get your puppy used to visits to the vet's office when they are still young, there is much you can do throughout the life of your adult dog that will help to keep these visits to a minimum. Be sure to read Chapter 8 (Care of the Happy English Springer Spaniel) that outlines many things you can do to help ensure your dog remains as healthy as possible.

Back to the pen and paper exercise.

When you pay attention, and take the time to think about the many things you can do that will keep your dog happy, even more ideas will present themselves along the way, and you and your chosen canine companion will enjoy a long and happy life together. Take my word for it, and *do make the time for this fun exercise* because you will thank me later.

In a Nutshell

The above paragraphs are a short synopsis of what I think makes for a Happy English Springer Spaniel, and I'm sure you may have many more ideas to contribute to this list.

The following Chapters of this book contain much more detail concerning what every conscientious English Springer Spaniel guardian needs to commit to, on a daily basis, in order to ensure that the human family and the chosen canine companion have the best opportunity for living a long, happy and healthy life together without ever having to experience any unwanted behavioral issues.

When you want to raise a Happy canine companion that is a joy to share your life with, you will want to carefully read through the entire coming Chapters, while always keeping in mind, not just what makes you and your family happy, but what makes your dog happy as well.

Chapter 3: Overview of the Happy English Springer Spaniel

"If I could be half the person my dog is,
I'd be twice the human I am."
— Charles Yu

I cannot stress enough how important it is that you understand the basics of any breed you may be considering sharing your life with, such as size, energy level, intelligence, temperament, and exercise requirements. Once you are familiar with the basics, you can truly understand if you are the right person or family for sharing your life with a particular dog.

When considering this companion for your family, keep in mind that this breed has been separated into working (field lines), or show lines, so you need to know what you want. As an example, a dog bred from the show dog gene pool would most likely lack the speed and stamina that makes the working field dog a successful hunter.

As well, a dog bred for hunting in the field will usually have a shorter, docked tail, shorter ears and a coat that is more wiry or coarse than the heavier show dog that has longer ears and a longer coat.

Learning about the temperament, health and where this dog's ancestors originally came from will help you choose wisely to ensure that your lifestyle and daily routine can meet this dog's needs.

History

This dog is a close relative of the English Cocker and Welsh Springer Spaniels. At one time both were born into the same litter, and the smaller cockers used to hunt Woodcock and the larger Springers used to flush game.

English Springers were officially recognized as a distinctly different breed over 100 years ago (1902) by the Kennel Club of England.

DID YOU KNOW? *The English Springer Spaniel is a sniffer dog used in many different roles and they are named for their original hunting role where they "spring" to flush birds from their hiding place so that they will take flight.*

Be aware that when you don't carefully choose a breeding line, some of these dogs can suffer from a sudden, frightening flare up of dominant or aggressive tendencies. You should never scrimp on socializing and teaching this dog firm rules and boundaries.

The versatile English Springer Spaniel learns quickly and responds well to positive training methods. They are eager to learn, and most make great watchdogs that will bark sharply at the door to alert you. As well, they tend to be polite and non-aggressive toward strangers and also peacefully accepting of most other dogs and household cats. A well-trained and socialized English Springer may be the perfect companion for the active family because they thrive on vigorous activity.

However, if you prefer a tidy home, this breed may not be the best choice for you because they shed and love getting wet, whether swimming, running through mud puddles and tipping over water bowls; this means that tracking hair, mud and debris through the house will be a common occurrence.

While the English Springer Spaniel temperament is usually polite and peaceful, if they are left on their own too much, they may display their unhappiness through destructive chewing, excessive barking or the development of separation anxiety.

Recognized by the American Kennel Club (AKC) in 1910, this athletic, friendly and versatile canine is a loving and eager to learn companion that currently holds the #27 popularity position amongst the 193 AKC registered purebreds.

OK, now that you have a basic understanding of the history of this versatile spaniel, following is the main overview of the breed, which will be the foundation of wisely choosing and raising a happy and well-behaved dog.

English Springer Spaniel Vital Statistics

While every dog is unique, there are standards that are common to each purebred canine, such as height, weight and various coat types, colors and features. You can also get a pretty good idea of what the puppies will look like when full grown, when you see their parents.

Height and Weight

When measured at the shoulder on average, this sturdy, medium-sized dog may stand between 17 and 20 inches (43 and 51 centimetres) and ideally weigh between 35 and 55 pounds (16 and 25 kilograms) or more or less, depending on the size of both breed parents, with an average lifespan of between 12 and 14 years.

Coat Colors and Common Features

Depending upon whether this spaniel is from a show line or a working field line, their features may be quite different from one another. For instance, the double coat of the working line spaniel will be medium length, flat or slightly wavy or wiry, with a short, soft and dense undercoat to help make the dog thorn and weather proof and also partially waterproof when outside working in the field. The show dog will have a thinner, silkier coat that will be longer.

The eyes are oval-shaped and varying with coat color from dark hazel to very dark brown or black. The long, feathered ears are medium size with rounded tips, and the nose color will vary between liver and black, depending on coat color.

Often this dog's tail will be docked, and acceptable coat colors include black and white, black, white and tan, liver and white, liver, white and tan, white and black, and white and liver.

How Smart is the English Springer Spaniel?

While every dog is surprisingly different even within the same breed, despite what some "experts" might have to say about it, you need to keep in mind that there are *"people smarts"* and *"dog smarts"* and that these two ways of rating intelligence are often widely divergent or in conflict with one another.

If you really want to rate your English Springer Spaniel's intelligence, based on what we humans think is *"smart"*, there is a book *("The Intelligence of Dogs")* written in 1994 by Stanley Coren, which has become the standard for rating the particular intelligence of different canine breeds.

While I can agree, in part, with some of the information contained in this book, I can also disagree. I have much personal experience with many breeds, and while I concur with the high smarts rating for the English Springer Spaniel, I have found that some dogs that are rated very low on the intelligence scale are also very smart in their own way.

Therefore, I caution you not to pre-handicap your dog's level of intelligence just because of something you may have read in a well-respected book, because each dog has their own unique set of talents and much of how they develop mentally is up to their guardian.

Coren judges canine intelligence of particular purebred canines based on three categories, as follows:

"Instinctive Intelligence – a dog's ability to carry out tasks it was bred to perform, such as guarding, herding, hunting, pointing, retrieving or supplying companionship."

"Adaptive Intelligence – how well a dog is able to solve problems on its own."

"Working/Obedience Intelligence – how quickly a dog is able to learn from humans."

The English Springer Spaniel is a very smart dog that will usually be eager to learn and easy to train. Coren places this thinking dog in the #13 position out of 138 listed breeds in the *"Excellent Working Dogs"* category.

Please keep in mind that there are always exceptions to every study and a particular breed's degree of intelligence is often related to their early upbringing and how they are trained.

I have had personal experience with this breed, and can tell you that they are indeed eager to please and quick to learn. When you use fair and positive training methods that involve treat rewards, this will be an intelligent, versatile and willing to learn dog that will be highly trainable.

When training a puppy, be patient, consistent and no more than 5 to 10 minutes each time. It's important to learn when enough is enough so your puppy doesn't become overwhelmed and simply zone out.

If this dog is misbehaving, it's most likely because they are bored and they haven't had enough exercise. This energetic dog needs something to do that stretches their mind and body, and if you don't provide them with consistent, daily, sufficient mental and physical exercise, this dog will become stressed and unhappy.

Make sure that your training involves fair, firm guidance and discipline and plenty of socializing from a young age, so that he or she will listen to your commands, respect the rules and boundaries you've taught, and trust and follow you as their leader.

FACT *Any humans that don't have the confidence and sufficient knowledge to properly socialize, establish and then consistently enforce proper rules will soon find themselves seated at the back of the bus.*

English Springer Spaniels are sturdy, agile athletes with great stamina that can excel in any sort of advanced training or obedience competition, where retrieving and jumping skills are required, or in Agility (obstacle course) competitions, where fast running is required.

Temperament of the English Springer Spaniel

The versatile English Springer Spaniel has a social and happy temperament often described as enthusiastic, active, friendly, obedient, loyal, and easily trainable.

This Springer loves the company of children and other pets and if there is a water source nearby, you can be sure they will find their way into it.

The English Springer is a constantly merry, always wagging friend who never tires and is always ready for the next adventure whether it be stalking birds in the back yard, running seagulls at the beach, or working in their true hunting capacity flushing birds out in the field.

While they will certainly bark to let you know someone is at the door, due to their friendly and social nature, they will eagerly invite everyone to come right on in, whether friend or foe.

The English Springer is a people-loving dog and they will not be happy being left alone for long periods of time, which can cause them to develop separation anxiety, which will only become worse if the dog is also not receiving adequate amounts of daily exercise.

Remember, this is originally a working breed of dog that is used to having a job to do, and if bored, understandably, they will show their unhappiness at being left alone and having nothing to do by engaging in obsessive chewing and barking. If you work long hours, this is NOT the dog for you.

Most English Springer Spaniels are sturdy, yet gentle dogs that are alert and faithful companions always eager for the next adventure. This dog may be a good choice for active families with older children who understand how to respect a dog's space. This dog could also be a great companion for older adults who have the energy, time and mobility required to provide the daily exercise and mental stimulation this energetic companion will need.

Keep in mind that a lonely English Springer Spaniel will soon be bored and if left alone in a back yard will most likely find a way to escape. Should your yard be truly escape-proof, they may bark their heads off until someone calls the police.

Unfortunately, sometimes people choose the English Springer Spaniel as a companion based on all the wrong reasons, including:

- those pleading eyes

- the beautiful patterned coat

- feeling sorry for a dog surrendered to the SPCA

- fond childhood memories of a neighbor's dog

- their sturdy, medium size

- their best friend has the same breed

- their enthusiastic and loving temperament

- the constantly wagging tail

To choose any dog as your companion based on these superficial criteria is a BIG mistake that you will soon regret. Rather, you need to consider the personality of this breed and their strong need for close contact with their human guardians.

When this dog is chosen for the wrong reasons, once the puppy cute factor has worn off, and the family gets busy with other areas of their life, the result will inevitably be an unhappy, frustrated and under-exercised, stressed dog that suffers from separation anxiety and will soon become unhealthily overweight.

Any dog that is routinely unchallenged by moderate daily activity and mental stimulation, especially a highly intelligent one that comes from a working background, may develop problematic behaviors and suffer from separation anxiety. Unwanted behaviors with a bored English Springer Spaniel can be many, and as an example may include:

- eating baseboards

- raiding the garbage

- chewing holes in walls

- destroying furniture

- excessive barking

- destructive hole digging that will turn your back yard into what looks like the latest lunar moonscape

- escaping the house or yard entirely

TIP *If you make the mistake of thinking your dog will be safe left to their own devices in your fenced back yard, and still be there when you return home, think again. You may be surprised at how determined this athletic companion is and what they will do to escape the back yard in search of something interesting to do.*

The English Springer Spaniel lives for their family and if left alone they will be very unhappy, which could encourage them to become a talented escape artist. The determined and intelligent English Springer Spaniel may figure out how to escape from confinement by using their strong legs to jump fences, climb fences, dig under fences or find cracks they can squeeze through if they want to get out. When this dog is bored and lonely, they usually <u>WILL</u> want to get out because they always want to be with their human family or engaged in some sort of interesting task or routine that challenges both body and mind.

When you have the right, active lifestyle and are able to keep this smart dog at your side throughout the majority of your days, and teach with a kind and consistent approach, he or she will be a highly trainable companion.

Every dog needs the discipline of being regularly walked on leash outside of the home each day, as well as the opportunity for off-leash time to run and play fetch or enjoy socializing with other dogs.

Although the temperament of an English Springer Spaniel (or any dog) will vary from dog to dog, and be somewhat dependent upon breeding lines and their first weeks with the breeder, as well as the human guardian who has trained and socialized them during the first few months of their life, generally speaking, this versatile, agile, active, and energetic breed displays a loyal and enthusiastic personality with an alert and loving temperament.

Proper socializing and teaching basic commands should begin at a young age for the smart English Springer Spaniel, who can begin to learn basic commands at eight to ten weeks of age.

When treated kindly and trained with positive reinforcement, this spaniel will have a zest for learning new things very quickly and will love the attention any sort of training program provides.

Always keep in mind that any dog, including the loving English Springer Spaniel, can become snappish if teased, provoked or is overly timid and afraid and feeling that it must fight back to protect his or herself. Therefore, without sufficient

socialization, a guardian should always be watchful when their dog is in the presence of younger, loud and boisterous children or feeling nervous around unfamiliar people, animals or circumstances.

Generally speaking, the personality of the English Springer Spaniel and how they develop will depend on whether they are bred from a social or antisocial line, and the skill of their human guardian when raising them.

BOTTOM LINE: this loyal dog will be happy so long as you engage them in moderate daily walks, high energy running free time, a vigorous canine sport, or perhaps spend time teaching him or her various tricks and routines.

The adult English Springer Spaniel is certainly capable of excelling at several canine sports, such as Agility, Flyball, Dock Diving, Field Training, Trick Training or Advanced Obedience.

Whatever you teach this dog, at a minimum, make sure that you always get them outside for several daily, 30-60 minute walks and allow them some off-leash time to run, swim, fetch and sniff or play with other dogs.

The highest priority for an English Springer Spaniel is always that they are kept busy by enjoying vigorous outdoor activities with their humans that exercise both their body and their intelligent mind.

When they are puppies, it's important to engage them in thinking and working activities because they need this stimulation as part of their on-going healthy development.

Just keep in mind that how active you are will have a sizeable impact on the health of your English Springer who will need to eliminate daily pent up energy by exercising their minds and their bodies so that they can remain a healthy weight. Remember that without sufficient daily activity this dog may soon become lethargic, overweight and unhealthy.

All puppies are energetic, including the English Springer Spaniel puppy, and if you are active with them at a young age, and engage them in training and activities that stretch their minds and bodies, chances are that they will continue to be active into their adult years.

On the other hand, if you are an inactive human, the chances are high that this dog will become lazy, overweight, bored and very unhappy, which can lead to unwanted behaviors and exacerbated health problems.

This is a social dog that may also suffer greatly from separation anxiety that may display how they are feeling by barking, destructive chewing or digging behavior in an attempt to escape their lonely confinement. The versatile English Springer can be just as happy living in a rural setting, or enjoying the city lifestyle, so long as their guardian gets them outside several times every day.

English Springer Spaniel Special Needs

The English Springer Spaniel is bred in two distinctively different lines (working or field, and show), so make sure you choose the right one.

This spaniel will require regular brushing to keep the feathered coat in good condition.

Without early and on-going socialization, plus choosing a stable breeding line, some of these dogs can suffer from an unpredictable, sudden and quite frightening display of aggression known as "rage syndrome".

As this energetic dog requires a moderate to high amount of daily exercise, if you have access to a bicycle, it may be a good idea to consider training them with a "Springer Bicycle Jogger" (**pictured**) that attaches to your bicycle, so they can receive a good amount of disciplined exercise in a short period of time, while still safely under your control.

The English Springer Spaniel lives for fun, interesting and challenging activity and being in close contact with their humans, which means that if you work outside of the home and cannot take this dog with you, or if you spend a lot of your life travelling where your dog cannot go, this may not be the companion for you.

What some humans don't take into consideration when considering this active breed is that they DO require being engaged in tasks that challenge them and at least a moderate amount of daily exercise. Keep in mind that making sure this dog is happy and contented may involve more time and attention than the average individual or busy family is able to provide.

While their high intelligence level, active, alert temperament and ability to solve problems on their own is what makes this dog so accomplished in many different areas, as well as an eager and playful companion in the right family, these are also the same features that in the wrong family make the English Springer Spaniel prone to quickly becoming bored and unhappy.

Keep in mind that this spaniel (even show lines) will likely retain some of their original flushing and retrieving urges, which means that this dog may display a desire to chase birds and small creatures. Depending on how strong this dog's hunting instinct may be, and how well trained they are, you may need to keep him or her on leash when out walking in areas where they could get into trouble.

Happy English Springer Spaniel Secrets

In 2004, Buster the English Springer Spaniel, who was a military detection dog during the Iraq War, received the Dickin Medal (the Victoria Cross for animals) for honored service that involved discovering a weapons cache hidden in a wall cavity that was covered by tin and behind a wardrobe.

The English Springer Spaniel was initially known as the *"Norfolk Spaniel"* after Dukes of Norfolk that were responsible for the creation of this breed.

The English Springer Spaniel has an excellent sense of smell and is often employed as a *"sniffer"* or *"detection"* dog to search out all manner of things, such as explosives, drugs, blood, bee nests, and more.

 A Springer named "Murphy" works at HM Prison Services in Norwich to find illegal mobile phones.

The English Springer Spaniel is also called simply the *"Springer Spaniel"*.

Over the years, many celebrities have shared their lives with the English Springer Spaniel, including two U.S. Presidents, Richard Nixon and George Bush, singer Elton John, and actor George Clooney.

The English Springer Spaniel is one of the oldest canine breeds still in existence today, with much speculation that they were around as early as 300 AD.

FACT ***As a result of this dog being bred to assist hunters with retrieving downed game, they usually retain a very strong retrieval instinct, which makes them excellent for playing fetch.***

This dog has energy to burn and lives to run, walk and swim, which means that if you are unable to commit to at least two hours of vigorous activity with this dog every day, he or she may become overweight, nervous and resolve to entertaining his or herself through destructive behavior.

If you'd like a super smart, active dog that can be a versatile companion, a hunting buddy or an enthusiastic competitor in the Agility or show ring, this blue ribbon champion could be the perfect dog for you.

In a Nutshell

Familiarizing yourself with the English Springer Spaniel breed, special needs, and early history, plus understanding their intelligence level, temperament and exercise requirements will help you to decide if this dog, that has been well loved by so many for a very long time, is the right companion for you and your family.

Obtaining a comprehensive understanding of the breed's needs will not only save you and your dog from much future grief, but it will be a prerequisite for raising a content, well-behaved, and happy dog that you are proud to call your best friend and companion.

Chapter 4: Healthy English Springer Spaniel = Happy Dog

"Dogs are not our whole life,
but they make our lives whole."
— Roger Caras

If your English Springer Spaniel is not physically healthy, he or she will not be a happy canine companion for very long, because suffering from health-related issues can easily create a miserable and ill-mannered dog.

It's prudent that you take the many steps outlined here to help ensure that you are doing all that you can to keep on top of your English Springer Spaniel's good health.

Make sure you take the time to choose a veterinarian that can provide yearly check-ups, have your dog spayed or neutered in a timely fashion, choose a healthy diet for him or her, and carefully read this section so that you educate yourself about issues that may adversely affect your dog's health.

As well, take the time to learn a little canine CPR, because doing so may save the life of your own dog, or someone else's.

Below you will find more information on each one of these steps you need to take to raise a healthy and happy dog.

Choose Your Veterinarian Wisely

Some clinics specialize in caring for smaller pets, while some specialize in larger animal care, and others have a wide-ranging area of expertise and will care for all animals, including livestock and reptiles.

Choosing a good veterinary clinic will be very similar to choosing the right health care clinic or doctor for your own personal health, because you want to ensure that your puppy or adult dog receives the quality care they deserve. A good place to begin your search will be by asking other dog owners where they take their furry friends and whether they are happy with the service they receive.

Take your Springer Spaniel into your chosen clinic several times before they actually need to be there for any treatment, so that they are not fearful of the new smells and unfamiliar surroundings.

Consider Timely Neutering or Spaying

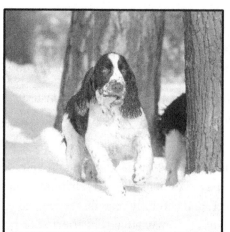

There are varying opinions on the topic of the best time to neuter or spay your young English Springer. One thing that many do agree upon is that earlier spaying or neutering, between 4 and 6 months of age, can be a better choice than waiting longer.

Keep in mind that non-neutered or spayed males and females are more likely to display aggression related to sexual behaviour, than are dogs that have been neutered or spayed.

For instance, fighting, particularly in male dogs that is directed at other males, is less common after neutering. The intensity of other types of aggression, such as irritable aggression in females will be totally eliminated by spaying, so make that appointment at the vet's office and get it done.

Effects on General Temperament: many dog owners often become needlessly worried that a neutered or spayed dog will lose their vigor, when in fact, many unwanted, aggressive qualities, resulting from hormonal impact, may resolve after surgery, and you will be acting as a conscientious, informed, and caring guardian.

Effects on Escape and Roaming: a neutered or spayed spaniel is less likely to wander, and castrated male dogs have the tendency to patrol smaller sized outdoor areas and are less likely to participate in territorial conflicts with perceived opponents.

Possible Weight Gain: while metabolic changes that occur after spaying or neutering can cause some puppies to gain weight, often the real culprit for any weight gain is the human who feels guilty for subjecting their puppy to this medical procedure, and in an attempt to make themselves feel better, they feed more treats or meals to their companion.

If you notice weight gain after neutering or spaying your English Springer Spaniel puppy, simply adjust their food and treat consumption as needed and once stitches are healed, make sure that they are receiving adequate daily exercise.

Educate yourself with respect to vaccination

It has now become common practice to vaccinate adult dogs every three years, and if your veterinarian is insisting on a yearly vaccination for your puppy, you need to ask them why, because to do otherwise is considered by many professionals to be *"over vaccinating"*.

Whether or not your dog actually needs a booster can be determined with a simple blood test at your vet's office, so be proactive, and ask for a blood test.

Puppies need to be vaccinated in order to provide them with protection against four common and serious diseases referred to as *"DAPP"*, which stands for Distemper, Adenovirus, Parainfluenza and Parvo Virus.

Approximately one week after your puppy has completed all three sets of primary DAPP vaccinations, they will be fully protected from those specific diseases.

Be Aware of the Health Conditions That May Affect Your Dog

While a healthy, happy English Springer Spaniel may live to be 12 to 14 years (on average), and with proper care, sufficient exercise, mental stimulation, and the best diet they may not suffer from any of the below noted health concerns, it is prudent to list all concerns possibly associated with this breed so that you have a clear understanding of problems that *"may"* affect your dog, including:

Hip Dysplasia (see picture): is a degenerative disease in which the hip joint becomes weakened due to abnormal growth. Depending upon the severity of the disease, treatment will involve medication or surgery. Screening of the parents cannot guarantee that puppies will not be born with this problem.

Dysplasia occurs when the bone slips out of its rightful place in the hip or elbow socket. When the bone is out of joint, it can cause the dog to limp or it might cause total limb lameness. Over time, the wear and tear on the joints can lead to painful inflammation, which may necessitate a surgical repair. In more mild cases, other treatment options include pain medications and anti-inflammatories.

Elbow Dysplasia: is a condition in which the head of the dog's femur fits improperly into the elbow joint socket. Factors that have an influence include nutrition, a dog's environment and the condition of the elbow sockets of its parents. Screening is recommended for breeding stock.

Obesity: the English Springer Spaniel is well known for being prone to weight gain, because if there is food out, they don't know when to stop, and they often do not get enough exercise when living with busy humans. This means that an under-exercised overfed dog will easily become obese. Obesity can lead to joint problems and heart disease.

Cardiomyopathy: is a disease of the heart that causes weakness in the muscle tissues and a subsequent enlarging of the heart, which can lead to heart failure.

Ear Infections: as a result of their long hanging ears, this dog is commonly prone to ear infection or inflammation. Therefore, guardians need to make sure that the ears are kept clean, dry and free of excessive hair growth.

Progressive Retinal Atrophy: causes degeneration of the retina, which is part of the eye. The retina is the part that senses visual information and sends it to the brain. Degeneration of this vital part of the eye eventually will lead to blindness and this disease usually appears between 3 and 5 years of age. A simple DNA test is available to determine (without waiting for symptoms to appear).

Cataracts (see picture): the English Springer Spaniel can suffer from cataracts that cause the lens of the eye to become opaque or cloudy, leading to blindness.

While this disease usually occurs in old age, it can also appear in a younger dog and treatment involves surgical removal.

Technically speaking, a cataract is an opacity that forms in the lens of the eye and it can partially or completely obstruct your dog's vision. Though cataracts are not painful, there is a slight risk that the cataract could slip out of place and float around the eye or it could become stuck in the tear duct, blocking fluid drainage.

Unfortunately, cataracts cannot be prevented, especially if it is a condition your puppy inherited genetically. If the cataract is caught while still in the early stages, however, your vet may be able to take steps to slow the progression and maybe even save your dog's vision. In some cases, a dog's vision can be restored by surgically removing the cataract, however, there is a fairly long recovery period for this kind of surgery.

Retinal Dysplasia: this eye disease appears as streaks or dots in the retina of the dog's eye, which can lead to blindness.

Glaucoma (pictured): this eye disease, which is usually caused by an increase of fluid pressure in the eye, can cause permanent damage to the dog's vision in the affected eye or eyes, which, if left untreated, can lead to blindness.

Entropion: is a condition in which the dog's eyelid will roll inward which then causes the lashes to rub against the eyeball. Left untreated, this condition can severely damage the dog's eye, even causing blindness. Surgery is required to correct this problem.

Hypothyroidism: is a condition resulting from an inadequate production of thyroid hormone and is treated with medication. Symptoms can include weight gain or obesity, constant hunger, reduced energy and a coarser feel to the dog's coat texture. Blood samples will be taken in order to test for a malfunctioning thyroid.

Epilepsy: is considered a neurological problem. The most common cause of seizures is idiopathic epilepsy, which is an inherited form of epilepsy. However, many factors can cause seizures and it is very important to have a dog diagnosed if seizures begin.

Phosphofructokinase Deficiency (PFK): this problem results from a recessive gene preventing the proper metabolizing of glucose into energy. A dog with this condition will be very low energy, preventing them from being able to exercise.

DNA testing is possible before breeding in order to prevent two dogs with the same recessive gene from producing puppies with this deficiency.

Deafness: inherited deafness affects quite a number of dog breeds. In most breeds, this is associated with white coat coloration around the head, as this is linked to the piebald and/or merle genes. Deafness usually occurs in puppies within a few weeks of birth and it can occur in only one ear, or both ears. There is no cure and puppies that are deaf in both ears are often euthanized because they are accident prone, startle easily, which can lead to biting, and can be difficult to train.

Bloat (Emergency Gastrointestinal Syndrome): is a life-threatening, common occurrence that can affect any deep-chested canine, and 50% of dogs that develop bloat do not survive. This condition can happen very quickly, especially if you feed your dog right after vigorous exercise, or if they are a very fast eater and gulp in large quantities of air with their food.

The stomach then distends with gas and fluid which can cause the stomach to twist 180-degrees or more. When the stomach is closed off, the food is then trapped inside where it will ferment and cause the stomach to bulge. The bulging stomach can then interfere with blood circulation and obstruct veins in the abdomen, which creates low blood pressure, followed by shock and damage to internal organs.

Bloat is a serious, life-threatening condition that requires immediate veterinary intervention. If you have a deep chested dog that tends to gulp their food, get them a slow feeder type of bowl to slow down their eating process and never feed them immediately after exercise or having had a large drink of water.

Rage Syndrome: is thought to be an inherited type of epilepsy, which appears as sudden, unexplained, violent attacks in a dog that is otherwise calm and well behaved. This usually does not display itself until the dog is approximately two years of age.

When you take good care of your happy English Springer Spaniel's health, and they come from a trusted breeder, he or she may never have to suffer from any of the above-noted list of health problems.

FACT *Most Springers will be particularly obsessed with retrieving balls and sticks. Do NOT use tennis balls because they are made with fiberglass, which will wear down your dog's teeth. Use only balls that are certified safe for dogs.*

Educate Yourself About Common Canine Diseases and Viruses

While your dog may never suffer from a common disease or virus, in order to ensure the safety and health of your happy English Springer Spaniel, you need to be aware of the many common diseases and viruses that could detrimentally affect the health of your dog.

Always watch out for the symptoms of the following common diseases and if you suspect that your dog has been infected, contact your vet immediately.

Distemper (sometimes called *"hard pad disease"*): is a contagious, serious, and deadly viral illness that is spread through the air or by direct or indirect contact with a dog (or other animal) that is already infected (such as ferrets, raccoons, foxes, skunks and wolves), that can also cause thickening of the pads on the feet or nose.

Early symptoms include fever, loss of appetite and mild eye inflammation that may only last a day or two, with symptoms becoming more serious and noticeable as the disease progresses. There is no known cure.

Adenovirus: causes infectious canine hepatitis, which can range in severity from very mild to very serious. The treatment focuses on management of symptoms, and the condition can sometimes result in death. Symptoms can vary and may include coughing, loss of appetite, increased thirst and urination, tiredness, vomiting and seizures.

Canine Parainfluenza Virus (CPIV): also referred to as *"canine influenza virus"*, *"greyhound disease"* or *"race flu"*, which is easily spread through the air or by coming into contact with respiratory secretions. While it is usually a self-limiting virus that will run its course within a couple of weeks, in severe cases and without antibiotic treatment, it may be fatal.

Symptoms can include a dry, hacking cough, difficulty breathing, wheezing, runny nose and eyes, sneezing, fever, loss of appetite, tiredness, depression and possible pneumonia. In cases where only a cough exists, tests will be required to determine whether the cause of the cough is the parainfluenza virus or the less serious *"kennel cough"*.

Canine Parvovirus (CPV): is a highly contagious viral illness affecting puppies and dogs, foxes, coyotes and wolves. Symptoms include vomiting, bloody diarrhoea, weight loss, and lack of appetite. Without prompt and proper treatment, dogs that have severe parvovirus infections can die within 48 to 72 hours.

Treatment will involve addressing dehydration and correcting electrolyte imbalances by administering intravenous fluids. Anti-inflammatory and antibiotic drugs are also given to control or prevent septicaemia, as well as drugs to control diarrhoea and vomiting.

Other Diseases and Viruses to Be Aware Of

What is Zoonotic? Zoonotic means a contagious disease that can be spread between both animals and humans.

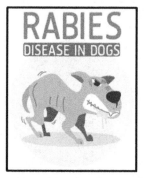

Rabies: is a viral, zoonotic disease transmitted by coming into contact with the saliva of an infected animal, usually through a bite. The virus travels to the brain along the nerves and once symptoms develop (usually marked by a change in temperament), after a prolonged period of suffering, death is almost certainly inevitable. There is no treatment.

In most countries, vaccination against rabies is mandatory between the ages of twelve and sixteen weeks. If you plan to travel out of State or

across country borders, you will need to make sure that your dog has an up-to-date Rabies Vaccination Certificate (NASPHV form 51) indicating they have been inoculated against rabies.

Leishmaniasis: is a contagious zoonotic infection caused by a parasite and is transmitted by a bite from a sand fly. While treatment involves the administration of a special drug (sodium stibogluconate), there is no definitive answer for effectively combating Leishmaniasis (especially since one vaccine will not prevent the known multiple species), with the prognosis often being fatal.

Symptoms include loss of appetite, diarrhoea, severe weight loss, exercise intolerance, vomiting, nosebleed, tarry feces, fever, pain in the joints, excessive thirst and urination, inflammation of the muscles, and death from kidney failure.

Lyme Disease: is one of the most common zoonotic tick-borne diseases in the world, which is transmitted by Borrelia bacteria found in the deer or sheep tick. Symptoms of this disease in a young or adult dog include recurrent lameness from joint inflammation, loss of appetite, depression, stiff walk with arched back, sensitivity to touch, swollen lymph nodes, fever, kidney damage, as well as rare heart or nervous system complications.

Control of the symptoms involves a lengthy course of antibiotic treatment in order to completely eliminate the organism.

Rocky Mountain Spotted Fever (RMSF): is a zoonotic disease transmitted by both the American dog tick and the RMSF tick, which must be attached to the dog for a minimum of five hours in order to transmit the disease.

Common symptoms include fever, reduced appetite, depression, painful joints, lameness, vomiting and diarrhoea, and some dogs may develop heart abnormalities, pneumonia, kidney failure, liver damage, or even neurological signs, such as seizures or unsteady, wobbly or stumbling gait. Treatment involves a 2-3 week course of antibiotics (Doxycycline or Tetracycline).

Ehrlichiosis: a tick-borne disease transmitted by both the brown dog tick and the Lone Star Tick, with common symptoms including depression, reduced appetite, fever, stiff and painful joints and bruising. The signs of infection typically occur less than a month after a tick bite and last for approximately four weeks. There is no vaccine available. Treatment involves a long course of antibiotics.

Anaplasmosis: deer ticks **(pictured)** and Western blacklegged ticks are carriers of the bacteria that transmit canine Anaplasmosis. However, there is also another form of Anaplasmosis (caused by a different bacteria) that is carried by the brown dog tick.

Because the deer tick also carries other diseases, some animals may be at risk of developing more than one tick-borne disease at the same time. Signs are similar to Ehrlichiosis and include painful joints, diarrhoea, fever, and vomiting, as well as possible nervous system disorders. Treatment involves administering the antibiotic Doxycycline for a 30-day period.

Tick Paralysis (pictured): this zoonotic infection is caused when ticks attach themselves to the skin and secrete a neurotoxin that affects the

nervous system. Affected dogs show signs of weakness and limpness approximately one week after being first bitten.

Symptoms usually begin with a change in pitch of the dog's usual bark, and weakness in the rear legs that eventually involves all four legs, followed by the dog showing difficulty breathing and swallowing. Your dog can die if not diagnosed and properly treated by removal of the tick.

Canine Coronavirus: this highly contagious intestinal disease, which is spread through the feces of contaminated dogs, while now found worldwide, can be destroyed by most commonly available disinfectants. Symptoms include diarrhoea, vomiting and weight loss or anorexia. There is a vaccine available, which is usually given to puppies, because they are more susceptible at a young age. This vaccine is also given to show dogs that have a higher risk of exposure to the disease.

Leptospirosis: is a worldwide zoonotic bacterial infection that can affect humans and many different kinds of animals, including dogs. If left untreated, there is potential for both dogs and humans to die from this disease.

The good news is that this virus is usually treated with antibiotics and supportive care, and because you can protect your dog with a vaccination, it makes sense to vaccinate against this disease if you and your dog live in an area considered a hot spot for leptospirosis.

Be Aware: Allergies Can Adversely Affect Your Dog's Health

You may be surprised to learn that dogs can suffer from allergies in much the same way that people can. Not only can the English Springer develop allergies to certain food ingredients, but he can also develop inhalant or contact allergies. The general signs of allergies include the following:

- Itchy red skin (**see picture below**)

- Itchy or runny eyes

- Licking the base of the tail

- Sneezing or coughing

- Ear infections

- Diarrhea

- Snoring from throat inflammation

- Chewing the paws

Some of the things that the English Springer Spaniel can be allergic to include grass, weeds, pollen, mold spores, dust, dander, feathers, cigarette smoke, prescription drugs, perfumes, and cleaning products. They can also be allergic to certain flea and tick products, so be very careful which one you choose. You should also never use products on your dog that are not designed specifically for dogs – this includes shampoo.

One of the most common complaints discussed at the veterinarian's office when they see dogs obsessively scratching, biting, licking and chewing at their skin or paws is possible allergies, and there can be many triggers. When you educate yourself, you can help ensure your English Springer Spaniel never has to suffer from allergies and can lead a healthier and happier life.

Environmental allergies: what many of us humans seem to forget is that our dogs can develop allergies to dust, chemicals, grass, mould, pollen, car exhaust, various forms of smoke, or flea and tick preparations, as well as allergies to materials such as wool or cotton, and chemicals found in washing soap or chemicals found in cleaning products you use around your home.

Visual symptoms are usually first noticed on the dog's stomach, inside of their legs, and at their tail or paws. Because many allergies are seasonal, our dogs will often be more affected in the spring or fall, with some airborne irritants inhaled by your dog resulting in coughing, sneezing or watery eyes.

Pay attention and if you think that your dog may have come in contact with an irritant found somewhere in your environment, first give them a cleansing bath, with the proper canine shampoo and conditioner.

Junk food allergies: *"True"* food allergies usually account for only about 10% of allergy problems in our canine friends.

Be aware that itching, chewing and chronic ear infections are not actually caused by food allergies, but rather are the result of a suppressed immune system, which is the result of your dog eating a low-quality diet. Food sensitivity issues can often be completely resolved by changing your dog's diet to a high-quality food that is more easily digested.

For instance, check food ingredients because far too many dog food products contain gluten ingredients that are common allergens to our fur friends, such as corn, wheat and soybeans. Become a label reader and ask questions, before you choose your dog's food.

Take the Time to Learn a Little Canine CPR

Of course, nobody wants to find his or herself in a situation where the life of their precious canine companion is put at risk. However, the reality is that accidents happen, and therefore knowing a little bit about how to help save your beloved furry friend is time well spent.

First of all, remember to handle an injured dog very carefully and gently. A dog that is traumatized, fearful or in pain, even one that is usually gentle, may lash out and try to bite.

Consider taking a class, because there are many animal CPR courses being offered these days through community educational systems or even online.

It's also a good idea to put together a canine first aid kit, both at home and in your vehicle, in case of emergencies, that includes the following items:

- ❧ Antiseptic Wash for wounds (hydrogen peroxide)

- ❧ Blanket

- ❧ Gauze Bandaging

- ❧ Kwik Stop styptic powder

- Medical Tape

- Nail Clippers

- Non-Stick Bandages for wounds

- Scissors

- Sterile Eye Wash

- Tick Twister

- Towel

- Tweezers

- Wash cloth

It would also be prudent to obtain a copy of the American Red Cross emergency techniques called *"Saving Your Pet With CPR"*, and familiarize yourself with the proper way to administer CPR to a dog.

Artificial Respiration Step by Step

If your dog becomes unconscious, depending upon what happened to them, they may stop breathing and if they stop breathing, they will go into cardiac arrest, when the heart stops beating and the dog dies.

However, after breathing stops, and before cardiac arrest, the heart can continue to beat for several minutes and this is when performing cardiopulmonary resuscitation (CPR) or artificial respiration can save your dog's life.

Step 1: place your dog on his or her side on a flat surface.

Step 2: check to make sure that your dog has actually stopped breathing by watching for the rise and fall of their chest and feel for their breath on your hand. Check the color of your dog's gums, because lack of oxygen will make them turn blue.

Step 3: check that the dog's airway is clear and there is nothing stuck in their mouth or throat by extending the head and neck and opening your dog's mouth.

If there is an object blocking their throat, pull the tongue outward and use your fingers or pliers to get a firm grip on the object so that you can pull it free from the dog's throat. If you cannot reach the object that appears to be blocking the dog's airway passage, you will have to use the Heimlich Manoeuver to try and dislodge it (see below).

Step 4: so long as the dog's airway is not blocked, you can lift their chin to straighten out the neck and begin rescue breathing.

Step 5: hold the dog's muzzle and close their mouth, put your mouth over the dog's nose and blow gently – just enough to cause the dog's chest to rise.

Step 6: wait long enough for the air you just breathed into the dog's lungs to leave before giving another breath.

Step 7: continue giving one gentle breath every 3 seconds as long as the heart is still beating and until your dog starts to breathe on their own.

Canine Heimlich Manoeuvre

If breath won't go in, the airway may be blocked. In this case, you will need to turn your dog upside down, with his or her back held against your chest.

Wrap your arms around the dog and clasp your hands together just below the dog's rib cage (since the dog is being held upside down, this will be actually above the rib cage, in the abdomen).

Using both arms, give five sharp thrusts to the abdomen, and then check the dog's mouth or airway for the object. If the object is visible, remove it, and give two more rescue breaths.

CPR Step by Step

If your dog's heart has stopped beating, then CPR must be started immediately and ideal would be to have one person performing the artificial respiration, while the other performs the CPR.

Step 1: put your dog on his or her side on a flat surface.

Step 2: feel for your dog's pulse or heartbeat by placing one hand over his or her left side, just behind the front leg.

Step 3: place the palm of your hand on your dog's rib cage over his or her heart, with your other hand on top of the first (for puppies, put just your thumb on one side of the chest and the rest of your fingers on the other side).

Step 4: press down and release, compressing the dog's chest approximately one inch (2-3 centimetres) and squeeze and release 80 to 100 times every minute.

While it's always the hope that you may never need to, if your dog is not breathing and there is no pulse, knowing what steps to take in an emergency (which includes how to do the doggy Heimlich Manoeuvre or apply compressions), could literally save the life of your own dog or maybe even someone else's.

In a Nutshell

While your dog may never suffer from any of the diseases or health problems known to affect this breed, you will want to know what *may* afflict your dog because being aware of the signs can help them live a longer life. As well, familiarizing yourself with emergency CPR procedures in the following American Red Cross chart could help you save your dog's life.

It is also prudent to take the time to choose a veterinarian that can provide yearly check-ups, have your dog spayed or neutered in a timely fashion and educate yourself about required vaccinations.

Taking the steps outlined in this Chapter will help ensure that your spaniel will always have the best opportunity to be healthy and happy throughout your lifelong journey together.

Saving your pet with CPR

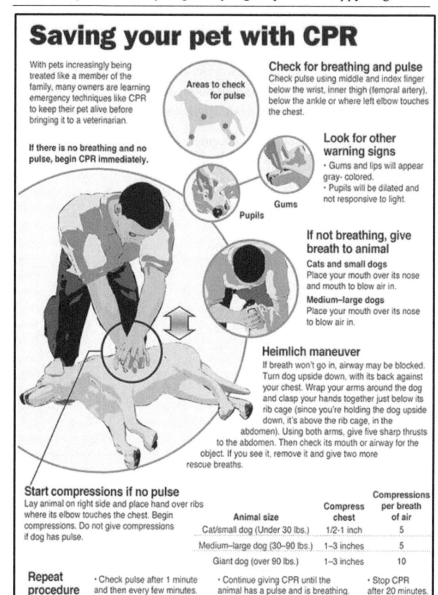

With pets increasingly being treated like a member of the family, many owners are learning emergency techniques like CPR to keep their pet alive before bringing it to a veterinarian.

If there is no breathing and no pulse, begin CPR immediately.

Areas to check for pulse

Check for breathing and pulse

Check pulse using middle and index finger below the wrist, inner thigh (femoral artery), below the ankle or where left elbow touches the chest.

Look for other warning signs

- Gums and lips will appear gray-colored.
- Pupils will be dilated and not responsive to light.

Pupils

Gums

If not breathing, give breath to animal

Cats and small dogs
Place your mouth over its nose and mouth to blow air in.

Medium–large dogs
Place your mouth over its nose to blow air in.

Heimlich maneuver

If breath won't go in, airway may be blocked. Turn dog upside down, with its back against your chest. Wrap your arms around the dog and clasp your hands together just below its rib cage (since you're holding the dog upside down, it's above the rib cage, in the abdomen). Using both arms, give five sharp thrusts to the abdomen. Then check its mouth or airway for the object. If you see it, remove it and give two more rescue breaths.

Start compressions if no pulse

Lay animal on right side and place hand over ribs where its elbow touches the chest. Begin compressions. Do not give compressions if dog has pulse.

Animal size	Compress chest	Compressions per breath of air
Cat/small dog (Under 30 lbs.)	1/2-1 inch	5
Medium–large dog (30–90 lbs.)	1–3 inches	5
Giant dog (over 90 lbs.)	1–3 inches	10

Repeat procedure
- Check pulse after 1 minute and then every few minutes.
- Continue giving CPR until the animal has a pulse and is breathing.
- Stop CPR after 20 minutes.

SOURCE: American Red Cross

Chapter 5: Let Your Dog BE a Happy Dog

*"Don't make the mistake of treating your dogs
like humans, or they'll treat you like dogs."*
— Martha Scott

This chapter is written to alert you to the fact that far too many of us humans have the tendency to treat our dogs more like human fur children than dogs.

You need to understand that not allowing your fur friend to be *"dog-like"* is very important when we're talking about THEIR happiness, because treating a dog like a human can ultimately result in <u>you</u> creating any number of behavioral issues.

<u>Your Dog is Not a Child</u>

While this might sound like a strange Chapter title, there is no doubt that many humans simply don't allow their dogs to actually BE dogs, because they are too busy confusing their dog by attributing human emotions to them, and treating them like children.

Today, the urge for humans to treat their dogs much more like children than dogs is becoming more and more of a serious problem. In reality, no matter the size of the dog, they need to be accepted as dogs. When you begin to expect your dog to fulfill an emotional void that can only be met by a human companion, you are embarking down a road that can lead to many problems for both of you.

Yes, some dogs may need to wear clothing to keep warm and dry, and depending on where they live, their guardian may need to provide them with protection from the cold and rain during the winter months. However, this is not usually the case with an energetic spaniel, and if the only reason you are dressing up your dog is because it makes you laugh, or appeals to a frustrated maternal instinct, this is NOT a healthy relationship.

Also keep in mind that if you live in a warm climate, you may want to provide your dog (especially one with a darker coat) with a cooling vest or a simple white t-shirt to reflect the heat during warmer summer months when they are walking outside in the sunshine.

When your English Springer is a full-grown adult, you will definitely want to begin more complicated or advanced training sessions. They will enjoy it and when you have the desire and patience and they have the willingness, there is literally no end to what you can teach this brilliant, eager to learn dog.

While some breeds of dogs of lower intelligence might be just fine without receiving daily interesting activities to keep them busy and mentally challenged, the English Springer Spaniel, with their high intelligence, lively and playful temperament, typically wants and needs to occupy much more of their guardian's time and energy by engaging in physical activities that also challenge them mentally.

A conscientious guardian of this breed will need to constantly be thinking of ways to challenge their bright and inquisitive canine companion and make their daily life interesting.

If you and your dog are really enjoying learning new tricks together, you might want to advance to teaching them the hand signals for *"commando crawl"*, how to *"speak"* or to *"jump through the human hoop"*, and depending on your particular dog, you may want to consider getting them involved in a fun canine sport, like Agility, Barn Hunt, Dock Diving, Trick Training or even get them certified as a therapy dog.

The only restriction to how far you can go with training your dog will be your imagination and their personal energy level, ability and desire to perform.

Every dog has a uniquely wonderful set of gifts to share with their human counterparts, if only us humans would listen. They *"tell"* us when they are unhappy, frightened, bored, nervous, and when they are under-exercised, yet often we do not pay attention, or we just think they are being badly behaved.

Many humans today are deciding to have dogs instead of children and then attempting to manipulate their dogs into being small (or large) furry children. This is having a seriously detrimental effect upon the health, happiness and behavior of our canine companions.

Single, lonely people often have dogs, which is just fine, so long as the human side of the equation doesn't expect their canine counterpart to fulfill what humans require on an emotional level, because this is very confusing to a dog who needs their human to lead them.

FACT *The English Springer Spaniel is not a breed well suited for the physically restricted or inactive or for humans that lead busy lives with long work schedules that keep them away from home. In order for this smart dog to be well balanced psychologically, they demand a lot of attention and will not be happy spending only a few minutes with their humans each day. This dog will also not be very happy leading a sedentary life because they have endless stamina and are highly energetic, curious and interested in what's going on around them and need to get out and about on a regular basis, rather than simply laying on the couch all day.*

In order to be the best guardians for our four-legged friends, we humans must have a better understanding of what our dogs need from us, rather than what we need from them, so that they can live in safety, harmony and security within our human environment.

Sadly, many of us humans are not well equipped to give our dogs what they really need and that is why there are so many homeless, abandoned and frustrated dogs and so many overflowing rescue facilities.

 As a professional dog whisperer who is challenged with the task of finding amicable solutions for canine/human relationships that have gone off the rails, I can tell you with certainty that once humans understand what needs to be changed and actually take the steps to do the work required, almost every stressful canine/human relationship can be turned into a happy one.

The sad part is that many humans are simply not willing or able to really understand the breed they are choosing, nor they are willing, able or honest enough about how much time they really have to do the consistent work and devote the time necessary to ensuring that their chosen dog's needs are truly met.

Almost ALL canine problems, both mentally and physically, are a direct result of incompatible energy and lifestyle. If you choose a dog without first seriously researching and being honest about your own lifestyle and how much time you truly can devote to a dog, you can almost be certain that problems will arise somewhere down the road. It's no secret that ignorance, time restraints or unwillingness on the part of the human guardian to choose the right dog and then learn what their dog truly needs will be a hit and miss undertaking that usually results in the "miss" coming out on top.

What we humans often forget to consider is that first and foremost, our dogs need to be respected for their unique canine qualities and we need to recognize how willing they are to bend themselves to our will so that they can fit into our human environment.

For millennia, dog has been considered *"Man's best friend"*. In today's society, when we want to do the best for our canine companions and create a harmonious relationship, we humans need to spend more time receiving the proper training WE need, so that we can learn how to be *"Dog's best friend"*.

Any dog can be your *"best friend"* providing that YOU educate yourself and put in the work. This is a universal truth that applies to any canine breed, including the active, faithful and highly intelligent English Springer Spaniel.

PERSONAL EXPERIENCE: Many times, I've been asked to come and correct "problems" in a family that has decided to share their lives with an energetic spaniel. They show me many pictures of destruction including a dug up back yard, torn apart couches and more and expect me to "fix" their unruly dog that is also disturbing the neighbors with their constant barking. In every instance, the poor dog is being blamed for being a sad, lonely, highly stressed and bored captive that needs something interesting to do, much more daily exercise, and just wants to be with his or her humans.

Rather than putting the blame where it rightfully lies, the humans expect this smart, sensitive and energetic dog to be happy living alone within the walls of a house while the family is away at work all day. Again, my pet peeve (no pun intended) flairs as I am forced to tell these people that what they have asked this dog to endure is just plain cruelty, and the all-day barking or itemized destruction is NOT the dog's fault.

While the dog is willing to change right away when they get what they need, for the humans it's a long road to set this type of situation right, and sadly many humans simply don't have what it takes or are not willing to admit that they have caused the problem. What follows is often yet another dog being abandoned and placed behind bars at the local SPCA. Choose wisely and please don't let this ever be your story.

If you're considering this very smart, loving and easily trainable dog for your family, be absolutely certain that you are able to involve him or her in interesting vigorous daily routines and tasks that will engage both their body and their mind while keeping this dog at your side throughout most of the day. Being the right person for this energetic, versatile, thinking dog will ensure that you are raising a happy dog that never has to suffer from behavioral issues or poor health.

In a Nutshell

It's important to understand that no matter the size of your chosen canine friend, you actually need to let your dog BE a dog if you want to raise a happy and healthy companion.

While being overly protective, babying them or treating them like a fur covered child may be something YOU need, it's not what THEY need, and can create much confusion that often will lead to behavioral issues sooner or later in life.

Chapter 6: Every Happy English Springer Spaniel Wants Exercise

*"The dog lives for the day,
the hour, even the moment."*
— Robert Scott

This breed will usually require a moderate to high amount of daily physical and mental exercise, that also includes going out for 2-3 on-leash walks, walking properly at your side (without pulling) every day. The smart English Springer Spaniel will also need space to run (or swim) freely and some challenging thinking tasks that exercise the brain. This varied combination will result in a strong bond of trust and respect between you and your dog that translates to both a healthy body and a healthy mind.

If you cannot commit to the time required to ensure your dog receives regular exercise each day, that engages both mind and body, this will soon be a very bored, overweight, unhappy, stressed dog that could develop multiple health and behavior issues.

Minimum Daily Exercise Requirements

- A minimum of three 30 to 60 minute, on-leash, disciplined walks outdoors where they are walking at your side without pulling, and paying close attention to your commands.

- A minimum of one hour running, swimming, romping and socializing with other dogs or performing an interesting canine sport.

- A minimum of 15 to 30 minutes every day teaching tricks, commands, hand signals or routines that will exercise the brain.

Once properly leash trained and heeding basic commands, the English Springer Spaniel will also need the reward of some off-leash freedom at a securely fenced local dog park where they can run, socialize, play with other dogs or perhaps fetch a ball or Frisbee and just enjoy being a dog.

When playing fetch, be careful that you do not teach your dog to swear at you or be disrespectful. You've seen it yourself I'm sure, or at least heard it. This is when a dog has been taught by their humans to be ball or Frisbee obsessed. When the dog and human arrive at the park you can already hear the dog barking at their human to throw the ball before they are even out of the vehicle.

Don't Let the Dog Be in Charge

If you do not take the time to curb a barking habit during play, you may have to endure a noisy problem that will be irritating to you and everyone else within earshot.

When playing a game of fetch, it may take only seconds for this canine Einstein to teach their humans that they are in charge of the game. Literally, if you are not aware of what you are "teaching", all it may take is one slip up. Once you've made this mistake, your dog may never forget, or correcting it may take a very long time. Your dog is excited to retrieve the ball or Frisbee, so he or she barks, and you immediately throw the desired object. Guess what? You just taught your dog to bark (or swear) at you to immediately get what they want.

To do nothing about your dog barking for what they want sends an unspoken message to him or her that you approve of this type of crazed behavior. If you simply laugh, thinking this is such a funny scene, you will be teaching your dog to continue to swear at you. Don't go there in the first place because reversing this problem can take many long and frustrating (not to mention noisy) hours to accomplish.

Instead, be proactive and teach your dog what is, and what is not acceptable. When you draw a firm line in the sand and are always consistent with enforcing rules and boundaries, you will have given your loyal companion the best opportunity for a happy and stress-free life.

The smart English Springer Spaniel can be stubborn and wilful because they are used to thinking for his or herself. This makes it even more important to always be consistent when teaching and enforcing rules and boundaries, which includes the proper way to greet other dogs. Your dog needs to know that YOU are always in control of what they do and will never permit any overly boisterous activity with other dogs or any attempt to dominate or chase other animals without your say so.

Keeping your dog "safe" first means teaching them rules and boundaries and then always being vigilant about enforcing them. For instance, if you are uncertain about another dog approaching, simply place yourself between your dog and the approaching dog until you are certain a friendly greeting will be the outcome.

Ideal Daily Exercise Requirements

A fully-grown English Springer Spaniel will be a playful, energetic and versatile dog with endless stamina that will excel when they receive a wide variety of fun and interesting daily mental and physical stimulation from disciplined walks, exercise, play and challenging mental games or canine sports.

This spaniel is a social, friendly companion who usually gets along well with everyone and is always eager for their next adventure at the side of their human family. Their skills are many, and they thrive on positive praise and physical affection. Get this fur friend involved in Advanced Obedience, Flyball, Dock Diving, Field Trials, learning to fly through an Agility course, or any number of other activities that will help to maintain a happy mental disposition and a healthy weight.

Keep in mind that, depending on the particular dog and how you raise him or her, they will generally be more or less energetic. This means that if you are more energetic and enjoy getting out for plenty of walks, energetic adventures, biking, hiking, swimming, participating in canine sports or play at the local park, your dog will grow up to enjoy these activities too. It's a simple formula: you are more energetic, your dog is more energetic and both of you will be healthier and happier.

 I've had English Springer Spaniel clients whose dogs were under-exercised, frustrated, bored, and overweight, and others whose dogs were super athletes whose days were filled with energetic athletic outdoor pursuits that kept both mind and body fit and healthy. In other words, if you're active, your dog most likely will be too, and truly, a non-active human should never be considering this dog for their companion.

There may be many sports and services appropriate for this multi-talented, athletic, smart and agile dog that include, but are not limited to:

- Obedience Competition
- Agility
- Rally Trials
- Trick Training
- Fast CAT
- Dock Diving
- Flyball, Frisbee or Disc Dog
- Canine Freestyle Dance
- Therapy
- Conformation Shows

This dog has great stamina and likes to run and retrieve, and a very good way to give them the amount of exercise they really need is to train them to jog beside your bicycle. Consider training this energetic spaniel to a *"Springer Bicycle Jogger" (pictured)*, so that they can receive a good amount of disciplined, vigorous exercise in a short period of time. You may find that you barely have to pedal and may wear out your breaks trying to slow down. Be sure never to overdo it, and always carry water for your dog.

The *"Springer Bicycle Jogger"* attachment for a bicycle is an ideal and safe way to adequately exercise this intelligent and energetic dog, while still keeping them under proper control so that they cannot chase after a bird, cat or other distraction.

The Springer easily attaches to any bicycle and the arm can be quickly removed when not needed. The large spring attaches to a harness on the dog and there is a quick release, break-away tab at the top of the rope in case the dog runs around one side of a pole while you and the bike are on the other side. As well, the large spring in this arrangement ensures that if your dog tries to lunge or chase a squirrel or other distraction, you and your bicycle will remain stable.

 The English Springer Spaniel is a loyal and loving dog that will bond very quickly with any and all family members in a very short period of time. A lonely dog will become depressed, anxious, nervous, timid or make his or her own entertainment by becoming destructive, noisy by barking all day long, or finding ways to escape and find something interesting to do.

Ideal Living Conditions for a Happy English Springer Spaniel

DOG GROOMING

"First, I want you to make sure that my dog is still in there someplace."

This versatile companion needs space to move and run and will not do well living in a rural setting where the living space is too confining. At the very minimum, this dog needs a larger home with a securely fenced back yard, plus the opportunity to get outside for their disciplined, on-leash walks, vigorous running, swimming, socializing and interesting tasks where they get to use their brain every day.

This athletic companion loves life and is always happy to head outside for the next adventure so long as it includes plenty of vigorous physical and mental activity in the company of their family.

Also, keep in mind that while this smart dog can sometimes be stubborn, the personality of every Springer will be different and each dog will develop traits and quirks that are unique to him or her.

How each puppy will develop will depend upon the breeding line, temperament of the parents, the environment where they are raised and how they are trained and socialized. The friendly, intelligent and eager to learn English Springer Spaniel will do best with a guardian that maintains firm rules and boundaries, and he or she will respond well to fair, firm and consistent training programs involving treat-based rewards or reinforcement.

Properly socializing at a young age, during the first three months of his or her life, will greatly influence the dog's adult temperament, personality and behavior as he or she matures, and will help to prevent this dog from becoming too bossy or manipulative. Continuing to shape the personality of this dog through adolescence and on into adulthood with proper socializing, training, plenty of exercise, and firm rules and boundaries, will help to ensure a well-mannered fur friend.

If you are unable to commit to providing the proper routine for this dog on a daily basis, that includes on-going socialization, training, mental games, and spending as much time as possible engaged in vigorous outdoor pursuits each day, this athletic dog will very likely first become unhealthily overweight, second, may become nervous around other dogs that can lead to fear aggression, and third, may become depressed.

An under-exercised Springer will soon become fat, bored and unhappy, which can then cause them to develop behavioral problems that could include acting out in destructive ways by chewing "off limits" items in the home, digging holes in the garden, escaping the back yard, excessive barking, and ultimately suffering from anxiety and stress that can prematurely cause health issues and shorten their life.

Above all else, never forget that all dogs (no matter their size) are pack animals, which means that it is not normal for them to spend long periods of time by themselves. This is even more important with a thinking dog that has a brilliant mind and comes from a working background, such as the English Springer Spaniel. Always remember that when you adopt a dog into your family you become their pack and you cannot simply abandon them, and forget about their needs when it's convenient for you to do so.

In other words, if you're planning to leave your companion alone for many hours every day, while you're at work or out for an evening at the pub with friends, ***PLEASE DO NOT*** get a English Springer Spaniel (or ANY dog for that matter); if you do, you will undoubtedly be contributing to your fur friend developing separation anxiety, a depressed, nervous and unhappy state of mind, and angry neighbors should your dog spend his or her lonely hours barking up a storm.

In a Nutshell

The bottom line here is that the English Springer Spaniel is an athletic, smart, thinking dog that lives for challenging activity while in the close company of their humans. This dog has great stamina and NEEDS plenty of interesting and fun activity every day.

So, even before you bring him or her home, start thinking about Advanced Obedience, Trick Training, Field Training, Dock Diving and many other canine sports, that should be in the future for this highly capable fur friend.

This Chapter outlines many different canine sports that this versatile dog may excel at, such as Agility, Flyball, or Freestyle Dance. Truly consider involving this dog in a sport, because this is a great way to provide them with the exercise they need in a disciplined way that will engage their thinking mind while keeping them slim and trim. These types of activities will help to ensure that your dog is a healthy and happy family member, while also teaching them that you are their leader.

Chapter 7: Feeding the Happy English Springer Spaniel

"I feel sorry for people who don't have dogs.
I hear they have to pick up food they drop on the floor."
— Unknown

It's not rocket science to grasp the concept that a properly fed dog means a healthy, happy and longer-lived companion, so make sure that you spend an appropriate amount of time to research high-quality food and treats that will be the best for your canine athlete and don't overfeed.

DID YOU KNOW? *This dog has a strong tendency to overeat. If there is food around, they do not know when to stop, so be careful not to overfeed or leave food items within their reach.*

We are what we eat, and the same is absolutely true for our canine companions. This breed usually has a very big appetite, and they will keep eating until all the food is gone, so practise portion control. Also, make sure that you don't get into the habit of *"doctoring"* their food bowl with your human food. If you do, your dog may soon refuse to eat their doggy dinner. Don't worry, though, because even a picky eater (which is highly unlikely with this foodie) will not starve him or herself, and if they refuse their expensive dog dinner tonight, so long as you don't cave, they WILL be hungry tomorrow.

First, remember that our canine friends are carnivores, which means that they derive their energy and nutrient requirements and maintain their health by consuming a diet consisting mainly or exclusively of the flesh of animal tissues. In other words, your dog is a meat eater.

Many dog owners underestimate the importance of feeding their dog a high-quality dog food and they make the mistake of shopping for dog food by price alone. The problem with this method is that the cheaper the dog food is, the poorer the quality. Inexpensive dog food brands use low-quality fillers and other ingredients to add bulk to the product, but these ingredients do not usually provide any nutritional benefit. Without a healthy, high-quality diet, your dog may not live as long as he or she could because poorly chosen food may lead to the development of health problems.

When choosing an appropriate diet for your English Springer Spaniel, considering the physiology of the canine's teeth, jaws and digestive tract will give you a better understanding of what food they should be eating.

Teeth, Jaws, and Digestive Tract

Teeth: canine teeth are all pointed because they are designed to rip, shred and tear into animal meat and bone. An adult dog has on average a third more teeth than his human guardian.

Adult canines have 42 permanent teeth in comparison to a measly 32 human teeth (without counting any wisdom teeth, which are "bonus"). Puppies have on average 28 baby teeth, while human babies will possess 20 "baby" teeth. Puppies start losing baby teeth at approximately 12 to 16 weeks of age. By four months of age, almost all of a puppy's baby teeth have been shed and many of the permanent teeth have already grown and are in place.

Jaws: every canine is born equipped with powerful jaws and neck muscles for the specific purpose of being able to pull down and tear apart their hunted prey.

The jaw of every canine opens widely to hold large pieces of meat and bone, while the actual mechanics of the canine jaw permits only vertical (up and down) movement that is designed for crushing.

Digestive Tract: the canine digestive tract is short, simple and designed to move their natural choice of food (hide, meat and bone) quickly through their systems.

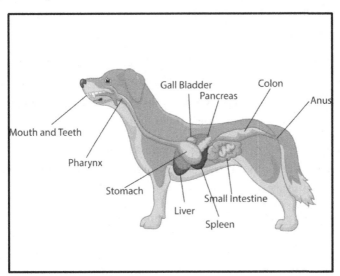

We humans need vegetables and plant matter in our diet and have the flat molars to effectively crush and chew them. While we often believe our dogs require the same, when choosing an appropriate food source for your English Springer Spaniel, you need to consider that vegetables and plant matter require more time to break down in the gastrointestinal tract. This in turn, requires a more complex digestive system that the canine body simply does not have.

The canine digestive system is unable to break down vegetable matter, which is why whole vegetables look pretty much the same going into your dog, as they do coming out the other end.

Consider how much healthier and long-lived your beloved English Springer Spaniel can be if, instead of largely ignoring nature's design for our canine companions, we chose to feed them whole, unprocessed, species-appropriate food.

Whatever you decide to feed your dog, keep in mind that, just as too much wheat or other grains and fillers in our human diet are having detrimental effects on our human health, the same can be very true for our dogs.

Read the labels so that you can be certain to avoid foods that contain fillers or high amounts of grains, because these are inappropriate for a healthy canine diet.

Also consider that even though dogs ARE carnivores, some do very well on a "plant based" diet simply because our meat sources are so often polluted with wheat, chemicals, drugs and other products that would not be part of a wild dog's natural diet.

As an example, one of the world's longest living canines was a highly energetic Border Collie who was fed a clean plant-based diet, and lived to be over 25 years of age, even though average for this breed is 14.

Control of Your Happy English Springer Spaniel's Food

Some dogs may be picky eaters, some may have a moderately healthy appetite, and others can be voracious eaters. The English Springer Spaniel most likely falls into the "voracious" category, and they can suffer from bloat from eating too quickly. *Get this dog a slow feeder type of bowl to slow them down.*

Any dog can get bored with eating the same food every day, so mix it up a little. For instance, my dog, Boris, usually has little interest in food during the morning, but is ready for his dental treat at high noon. His internal clock is spot on and if I'm not paying attention to the time, he just calmly sits there staring at me until I get it.

It's important that your dog understands that YOU are in control of their food source. Once they understand this, they will also figure out that there will be windows of opportunity for receiving and eating their food, and this routine will help to develop healthy eating habits.

Another crime that only CSI could solve.

Many people use a scoop or measuring cup to put dry food into their dog's bowl. This is a mistake, because it's very important to mix your dog's food with your hands, so that your scent is all over the food, before you give it to them to eat. This sends a "message" to your dog that you are their pack leader, because it mimics what would happen if you were the alpha dog out hunting for your food in the wild.

For instance, while a pack of wild dogs hunting for food all work hard to capture their prey, the alpha pack leader always gets to eat first while all the other dogs must wait until the leader of the pack eats their fill, before they can rush in to eat what is left over.

Therefore, when you are mixing your domesticated dog's dinner with your hands, you are sending them the subtle message that you are the pack leader, you've already eaten your fill and you are now allowing them to eat what was left over.

Nutritional Needs of the English Springer Spaniel

Before you go shopping for dog food take the time to learn the basics about the nutritional needs of your dog. Dogs are primarily carnivorous animals, which means that most of their nutritional needs should come from animal sources – including meat, fish, and eggs. Your dog needs a balance of protein and fat in their diet, plus healthy carbohydrates that can provide energy, fibre and other essential nutrients. It is important that your dog's daily food provides for their basic nutritional needs, because that is what he or she will be eating most of the time.

If you want to get into the specifics, know that protein is the most important nutrient for a dog and is required for healthy puppy growth and development. When your puppy grows up, protein will help him or her maintain lean muscle mass, so they do not become overweight or obese. Your puppy needs at least 22% protein in their diet and an adult dog needs 18%.

Next to protein, the most important nutrient for dogs is fat. While you may think of fat as a bad thing, it's actually an essential part of a balanced diet for dogs. Fat provides a concentrated source of energy and it helps your dog absorb and utilize fat-soluble vitamins. Fat should come from healthy animal sources such as chicken fat or salmon oil and should make up at least 8% of your young dog's diet. An adult dog will require a minimum of 5%.

Technically speaking, dogs do not have specific requirements for carbohydrate in their diet. Carbs can provide energy and they contain fibre as well as other nutrients.

What you also need to remember is that your dog's body is not optimized for digesting and absorbing nutrition from plant products as much as from animal products, which means that carbohydrates in your dog's diet should be limited. They should also come from easily digestible sources like whole grains, starchy vegetables, beans, or legumes.

Choosing a High-Quality Dog Food Brand

When shopping for food for your English Springer Spaniel, you need to take the time to carefully read the information on the package so that you can determine the quality of the product.

Also, if you're going to make comparisons between different products, there are three specific things to look for on the label.

AAFCO Statement of Nutritional Adequacy

First, look for the Association of American Feed Control Officials (AAFCO) statement of nutritional adequacy. This is an organization that sets and upholds standards for pet food and animal feed. If you and your dog live in the UK, check for information from the Food Standards Agency (FSA).

Before a product hits the shelf, these organizations examine it to make sure it meets the minimum nutritional requirements for the intended animal, which, in this case, is your dog. If the product is nutritionally balanced for dogs, you will see a statement like this somewhere on the label:

"[Product Name] is formulated to meet the nutritional levels established by the AAFCO Dog Food Nutrient Profiles."

If you see this on the package, you can rest assured that it will meet your dog's minimum nutritional needs. Keep in mind, however, that the AAFCO statement does not guarantee quality – you still have to read the ingredients list noted on the package to determine whether the product is any good or not.

Guaranteed Analysis

After the AAFCO statement, look at the guaranteed analysis – this tells you the percentages of protein, fat, fibre and moisture in the product. You can use the guaranteed analysis to make a direct comparison between products using those minimum values from the last section. Because your dog is better able to digest meat than plant foods, try to keep the fibre content less than 5%.

Ingredients List

After checking the guaranteed analysis, the final place to look is the ingredients list.

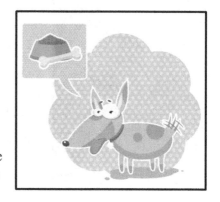

The ingredients list is ordered in descending order by volume, which means that the ingredients at the top of the list are used in the highest quantity – this is the same for packages of food that you eat. You will want to see healthy, high-quality ingredients at the beginning of the list starting with a source of animal protein. Dogs are carnivores, which means that their bodies are better able to digest and absorb nutrition from animal sources. Quality sources of animal protein for dogs include poultry, meat, and seafood.

Aside from proteins, fats, and carbohydrates, there are some other beneficial ingredients you can look for. Supplemental vitamins and minerals can improve your dog's health, because they help to ensure that your dog's specific nutritional needs are met.

DID YOU KNOW? *Synthetic supplements are not as good for your dog as natural sources for the same nutrients – things like fresh fruits and vegetables. When it comes to mineral supplements, chelated minerals are ideal – these are minerals that have been bound to protein molecules, which make them easier for your dog's body to utilize. If you see "dried fermentation products" on* *the list, do not be alarmed – these are probiotics that can support your dog's digestion.*

Feeding Tips

- ❧ Feeding amounts for canines vary based on factors such as breed, lifestyle, and body condition.

- ❧ While feeding suggestions are provided on all dog food packaging, your vet may be the best resource for telling you exactly how much you should be feeding your dog. See next section for generic feeding amount guidelines.

- ❧ Consult your vet regularly about your puppy's weight as achieving and maintaining an ideal weight not only reduces many health risks, but can also help your puppy have a more energetic, longer and healthier life.

- ❧ Do not overfeed! Numerous studies showed that dogs whose diets were responsibly restricted early on experienced longer lifespans and later onset of problems like osteoarthritis.

- ❧ If you give your dog the occasional treat or if you use treats for training, always remember to take this into account and reduce the daily food allowance.

- ❧ As a rule of thumb, treats shouldn't make up more than 10% of your dog's daily calorie intake as this can unbalance his diet.

- ❧ Although it's tempting and convenient to feed your puppy table scraps, they do not provide your pup with the correct balance of nutrients.

- ❧ A puppy or adult dog rarely says no to food, but that does not mean they are always hungry. Constantly giving them food can lead to unwanted behavior problems such as "begging for food" and hyper activity whenever they see you eating. Dogs are hard wired to always be foraging and looking for food and no matter how much you feed them, they will still ask for more. Therefore, make sure you don't let them develop this bad habit of begging for food.

❧ Any time you change your dog's diet, be sure to mix a little of the old food with the new food to transition them slowly – this will help to prevent digestive upset.

❧ If you mix your dog's food properly and he or she is still having digestive issues, it could be something else – such as food allergies.

❧ Food allergies affect dogs in a different way than they affect humans. While you might feel nauseous or sick after eating something you are allergic to, your dog will be more likely to develop skin problems, or throw up what they just ate.

❧ Red, itchy, and inflamed skin is a common sign of food allergies.

❧ Technically, your dog can develop an allergy to any food he or she eats, but there are some ingredients more likely to trigger food allergies in dogs than others.

❧ Some of the most common food allergens for dogs include beef, chicken, dairy, lamb, fish, corn, eggs, wheat, and soy, and this is usually because they came from food sources that are not "clean" or "organic". For instance, unless the chosen food is certified organic, grass fed and contains no additives, there are hidden components that can cause allergic responses. Crops such as corn, soy or wheat are often sprayed with chemicals and fed to farmed animals to fatten them up. This means that your dog may not be allergic to beef, but may be allergic to the wheat, soy or corn that's been fed to the animals.

🐾 If you suspect that your dog has a food allergy, you may need to put him or her on an elimination diet for 12 weeks or until all signs of the allergy have disappeared. At that point you can either keep feeding the elimination diet or switch to a food that doesn't contain the allergen.

Feeding Puppies

A general rule of thumb for growing English Springer Spaniel puppies is to feed daily amounts of between 2 and 3% of what the puppy's adult weight is projected to be or 10% of the puppy's current body weight. You will want to keep in mind that while all puppies require extra protein to help them develop into healthy adult dogs, this is especially important with higher energy puppies.

You will also want to keep a close eye to make sure that your puppy is eating and drinking enough throughout the day, so set regular feeding times each day. The smaller the puppy, the more important this will be.

There are now many foods on the market that are formulated for all stages of a dog's life (including the puppy stage). Whether you choose one of these foods or a food specially formulated for puppies, they will need to be fed smaller meals more frequently throughout the day (between 3 and 5 times), until they are at least one year of age.

As your puppy is growing, he or she needs more nutrients and calories than an adult dog, which is the reason why puppy foods have higher levels of protein and fat to support growth, as well as some nutrients like DHA, an omega fatty acid found in mother's milk. Once your puppy reaches adulthood, he or she doesn't need as many calories. Rich puppy food can quickly lead to excessive weight gain for adult dogs, so the transition to adult food is important.

English Springer Spaniels can be considered adults after about a year. They may still be growing after this time, but at the 12-month mark you can start feeding your dog adult food.

Feeding Adults

Choose foods that list high-quality meat protein as the main ingredient and, depending on your dog's particular energy level, feed between 2 and 3% of their body weight every day. While some dogs prefer one meal a day, most will appreciate morning food (after a walk) and evening food (after a walk).

Be careful not to get caught up in "convenience" when you're out grocery shopping for yourself, and decide to buy your dog's food at the same place, because most grocery stores tend to carry inferior brands of dog food.

Instead, make the time to visit your local pet store, talk with educated representatives, avoid grains, and choose quality sources of meat protein for healthy puppies and dogs, including beef, buffalo, chicken, duck, fish, hare, lamb, ostrich, pork, rabbit, turkey, venison, or any other source of wild meaty protein.

Treats

There are endless choices of dog treats lining the shelves of every feed store, pet store, and grocery store, and it will be an overwhelming task to choose wisely, unless you keep one simple rule in mind, and choose treats that contain only one ingredient or very few ingredients.

Whatever reason you choose to give treats to your English Springer Spaniel, keep in mind that if we treat our dogs too often throughout the day, they can become overweight, and we may create a picky eater who will no longer want to eat their regular meals. Think about it – if you got to eat only your favourite tasty treats throughout the day, would you be excited about consuming a less flavourful meal come dinner time?

DID YOU KNOW? *Researchers in Sweden have discovered that dogs were happier when they had to* <u>*earn*</u> *their treats as a reward for completing a task, rather than just being given a treat for looking cute, because just like us humans who get that happy "eureka" moment when we finally solve a problem, the same is true for our canine counterparts. The English Springer Spaniel is the perfect dog for positive training methods that involve treat reinforcement.*

Dangerous Treats

Always carefully read labels and take note of where treats are manufactured, because not all countries have the most stringent manufacturing protocols, and honestly there are many treats that you absolutely should NOT be feeding to your dog even though he or she may like them, including:

Rawhide (pictured) is soaked in an ash/lye solution to remove every particle of meat, fat and hair and then further soaked in bleach to remove remaining traces of the ash/lye solution. Now that the product is no longer technically food, it no longer has to comply with food regulations.

The wet rawhide is shaped into chews, and once dry it shrinks to approximately 25% of its original size before arsenic-based products are used as preservatives, and antibiotics and insecticides are added to kill bacteria.

While rawhide chews are tough and long lasting, when a dog chews a rawhide treat, they ingest many harsh chemicals. Also, when your dog swallows a piece of rawhide, that piece can swell up to four times its size inside your dog's stomach, which can cause anything from mild to severe gastric blockages that could become life threatening and require emergency surgery. As much as it might be convenient for you to be able to give your dog or puppy a treat that will occupy them for a considerable time, if it's rawhide, just say "NO".

Pig's Ears (pictured) are very attractive to most dogs that will eagerly devour them, and they're "natural" because they're ears, so what could be wrong? Actually, these are thin, crispy and very high in fat, which can cause stomach upsets, vomiting and diarrhoea. In addition, pieces can break off and become stuck in a dog's throat or cause perforations in the mouth, throat or digestive tract.

Also, pig ears are often processed and preserved with unhealthy chemicals that discerning dog guardians will NOT want to feed their dogs. Just say "NO".

Hoof Treats (pictured) are actual cow, bison, horse and pig hooves that humans believe are healthy, *"natural"* treat choices for their dogs when the truth is that after processing with harsh chemicals, preservatives and antibiotics, they retain little, if any, of their *"natural"* qualities.

Also, hooves are very hard and can cause the chipping or breaking of your dog's teeth as well as perforations in the mouth, throat or intestines, or blockages in your dog's intestines. Again, just say "NO".

Healthy Treats

As there are so many healthy treat choices available, honestly there's no excuse for feeding your dog unhealthy, toxic, nutrient-deficient or dangerous treats that could harm them. Read the labels to make sure the treats you are choosing are appropriately sized for your dog and are of the highest quality. Examples of healthy treats include:

Hard Treats: come in many varieties of shapes, sizes and flavors and will help to keep your dog's teeth cleaner.

Soft Treats: are also available in endless varieties and flavors, suitable for all the different needs of our furry friends and are often smaller in size and used for training purposes.

Dental Treats or Chews (pictured): are designed with the specific purpose of helping your dog to maintain healthy teeth and gums by exercising the jaw and massaging gums, while removing plaque build-up near the gum line.

The very best thing you can do for your dog's oral hygiene is to brush his or her teeth every day or two. However, dog dental chews can be an excellent top-up between brushing or for dogs who will not let you get anywhere near their teeth without a great struggle.

Dental chews come in both edible and non-edible varieties and lots of dogs love the taste of these chews and think of them as a tasty treat. Non-edible chews are a bit like toys for many dogs and satisfy their natural urge to chew while helping to clean their teeth at the same time.

Freeze-Dried and Jerky Treats (pictured): offer a tasty morsel most dogs find irresistible as they are usually made of simple, meaty ingredients, such as liver, poultry and seafood. Be careful when choosing jerky treats, as they are often processed with too much salt.

Human Food Treats: be very careful when feeding human foods to dogs as treats, because many of our foods contain unhealthy additives, such as salt, sugar and other ingredients that could be toxic and harmful.

Also, educate yourself about the common human foods that are actually poisonous to our canine friends, such as grapes, raisins, onions and chocolate, to name a few.

Generally, the treats you feed your dog should not make up more than approximately 10% of their daily food intake, so make sure the treats you choose are high quality, with single or few ingredients so that you can help to keep your dog both happy and healthy.

The Right Food for Your Happy English Springer Spaniel

"Dog Food" has significantly changed since 1785, when the English Sportman's Dictionary described the best diet for a dog's health in an article entitled *"Dog"*. This article indicated that the best food for a dog was something called *"Greaves"*, described as "*the sediment of melted tallow made into cakes for dogs' food*".

From these meager beginnings, commercially manufactured dog food has become a massively lucrative industry that has only fairly recently evolved beyond feeding our dogs the dregs of human leftovers, because it was cheap and convenient for us.

Even today, the majority of dog food choices often have far more to do with being convenient for humans to store and serve, than it does with being a diet truly designed to be a nutritionally balanced, healthy food choice for our canine companions.

Educating yourself by talking to experts and reading everything you can find on the subject, plus taking into consideration several relevant factors, will help to answer the dog food question for you and your dog.

For instance, where you live may dictate what sorts of foods you have access to, while other factors to consider will include the particular requirements of your dog, such as their age, energy and activity levels.

Our dogs are also suffering from many of the same life-threatening diseases that are commonly found in our human society (heart disease, cancer, diabetes, obesity). These diseases all have a direct correlation with over-feeding and/or eating genetically altered foods that are no longer pure, in favor of a convenient, processed and packaged diet that is quick and easy for us to serve.

The Raw Diet: raw feeding advocates believe that the ideal diet for their dog is one which would be very similar to what a dog living in the wild would have access to while hunting or foraging.

These canine guardians are often opposed to feeding their dog any sort of commercially manufactured pet foods, because they consider them to be poor substitutes, and for the most part, I would agree.

For instance, many guardians of high energy, working breed dogs will agree that their dogs thrive on a raw or BARF (Biologically Appropriate Raw Food) diet and strongly believe that the potential benefits of feeding a raw dog food diet are many, whether your dog is earning a daily working wage or simply being your loyal companion, including:

- 🐾 Healthy, shiny coats
- 🐾 Decreased shedding
- 🐾 Fewer allergy problems

- Healthier skin

- Cleaner teeth

- Fresher breath

- Increased energy levels

- Improved digestion

- Smaller stools

- Strengthened immune system

- Increased mobility in arthritic pets

- Increase or improvement in overall health

A raw diet is a direct evolution of what dogs ate before they became our domesticated pets and we turned toward commercially prepared, easy-to-serve dry dog food that required no special storage or preparation.

The Dehydrated Diet (pictured): is available in both raw and cooked meat forms, which are usually air dried to reduce moisture and inhibit bacterial growth. While the appearance of dehydrated dog food is very similar to dry kibble, the typical feeding methods include adding warm water before serving, which makes this type of diet both healthy for our dogs and convenient for us to serve.

Dehydrated recipes are made from minimally processed fresh, whole foods to create a healthy and nutritionally balanced meal that retains more of the overall nutritional value, and will meet or exceed the dietary requirements of a healthy canine.

A dehydrated diet is a convenient way to feed your dog a nutritious diet, because all you have to do is add warm water and wait five minutes while the food re-hydrates so your dog can enjoy a warm meal.

The Kibble Diet (pictured): there is no mistaking that the convenience and relative economy of dry dog food kibble, which had its beginnings in the 1940's, continues to be the most popular pet food choice for many dog-friendly humans. Thankfully, there are now many high-quality kibble foods available.

The Right Bowl for the English Springer Spaniel: there are many different types and categories of dog bowls, including Automatic Watering, Elevated, Ceramic, Stoneware, No Skid, No Tip, Slow Feeder, Stainless, Wooden and Travel Bowls.

Always purchase bowls that are appropriately sized for your particular dog, and consider an elevated dining table **(pictured)** so that their head is up from the floor when eating and drinking.

Also, if your dog wolfs their food, or has a deep chest (like the English Springer Spaniel), consider a slow feeder type of bowl **(pictured)** to help slow down the speed at which they consume their food, so that they are not at risk for life-threatening bloat.

In a Nutshell

While food and treat choices for your favorite furry English Springer Spaniel can be overwhelming, a basic understanding of canine physiology and making wise decisions concerning all the many different types of food and treats available, will help you to add many healthy and happy years to your dog's life.

You are the sole protector of your canine companion, and I cannot stress strongly enough the importance of a well thought out choice when deciding what brand and type of food and treats you will feed your loyal canine companion.

Appropriate food/treat choices and being careful to not overfeed, may not only increase the length of your dog's life by avoiding unwanted health conditions, such as allergies, obesity, high blood pressure or bladder stones, good food choices will also provide your dog with optimal health so they can feel good and live a happy life!

Chapter 8: Care of the Happy English Springer Spaniel

"When you adopt a dog, you have a lot of very good days, and one very bad day."
— W. Bruce Cameron

Imagine you're travelling by car on a daily basis without being protected by a seatbelt or an airbag. How safe would you feel? Unfortunately, this is the reality for far too many of our furry friends, because their guardians have neglected their safety responsibilities.

Now, imagine going for months without washing your hair, cutting your nails or brushing your teeth. Again, that is the reality for many dogs, because their owners have not been advised with respect to the importance of good grooming. How happy and well behaved do you think such an ill cared for dog would be?

The following few paragraphs outline safe travelling, licensing, insurance and grooming requirements, all of which can help to ensure that your English Springer Spaniel is safe, legal and better cared for at the vet's office.

Keep in mind that if your dog is safely secured when travelling, they might not be dead or seriously injured should you be involved in a vehicle accident. We humans wear seatbelts to be safe – what about safety for our best fur friends?

Further, if your dog is properly licensed, they will be returned to you should they go missing, and this is a much happier dog than one spending who knows how long behind bars at a rescue or SPCA.

As well, if you have pet health insurance, chances are that your dog will be better cared for at the vet's office, which means a healthier and happier companion.

Tips for Keeping Your Dog Safe

Not So Safe Harness Restraints: is your canine companion safe when buckled into a safety harness for travel in vehicles? Be aware that many of the dog harnesses in the marketplace have a 100% failure rate.

If you cannot find a safety harness that has actually been strength and crash tested (i.e. optimal choice), the safest travel arrangement for any dog is to secure them inside a kennel, that is bolted to the floor or secured with the vehicle's seatbelt. Remember that a dog travelling in the front passenger seat, even one secured with a proper safety harness, may still sustain injuries (and even death) if the 100 mph force of the airbag strikes them.

Kennels: a dog kennel or crate will easily fit on the back seat of most vehicles and can be secured with the vehicle's restraint system. An English Springer Spaniel (or any dog) riding inside a kennel that is secure inside your vehicle will have the best protection in the case of a rollover accident, plus you will avoid the fines some locations are now levying for allowing a dog to roam freely inside a moving vehicle.

Air Travel: while the English Springer Spaniel puppy will usually be small enough to fit into a soft Sherpa bag for travel inside an airplane cabin (as carry-on baggage), they will soon be too large when they attain their adult size. Any puppies or dogs that are too large to fit comfortably inside a Sherpa travel bag will need to be transported inside a heated cargo hold.

Licensing: when you purchase your dog a yearly license or identifying tag that you attach to their collar, they will be legal, and should they become lost when wearing a license, there is a much higher possibility that your dog will be returned to you, instead of spending their last few days behind bars at the local SPCA or rescue facility.

Pet Health Insurance: purchasing health insurance for your dog means that they will usually live a longer, healthier and happier life, because they will receive better care throughout their lifetime.

Be aware that it's a better idea to begin insurance when your dog is a young puppy, because waiting until they are older will mean that your monthly premiums will be considerably higher.

Puppy Proofing

As a dog owner, it is your responsibility to make sure that your dog's needs are taken care of. It all starts with prepping your home for a new puppy by puppy-proofing to keep him or her safe. Next, you will need to learn what to feed your puppy and when to transition them to an adult dog food formula (previous chapter). You will also need to take care of your dog's grooming requirements, which is discussed later on in this chapter.

When it comes to preparing your home for a new dog, you will need to do some puppy proofing. Start by walking through your home and try to view it through a puppy's eyes to identify potential dangers. Here's a list of some of the things you may need to do:

- Store cleaning products where your puppy cannot reach them or put them in a locked cabinet.

- Put all trash in a can with a tight-fitting lid or keep it secured in a cupboard.

- Store open food containers in your pantry or cupboards – anything left out needs a lid.

- Tie up or bundle any electrical cords and blind cords so your puppy cannot chew on them.

- Pick up small objects from the floor – they are a choking hazard for dogs.

- Cover open bodies of water (such as the toilet, bathtub, outdoor ponds, swimming pools, etc.).

- Put all medications and other toiletries where your puppy cannot reach them, such as in the medicine cabinet and use childproof bottles.

- Make sure none of your houseplants or plants in your yard are toxic to dogs – if there are any suspect plants or flowers, remove them, move them out of reach, or fence them off.

- Keep your windows and doors securely closed when your puppy is out – use baby gates or pet gates to keep them away from areas where you do not want them to wander.

- If you have a cat, keep the litter box where your puppy cannot reach it, so he does not eat the clumps.

❧ Dispose of all food waste properly so your puppy cannot get it – this is especially important for chicken bones and foods that are harmful to dogs.

❧ Store all lawn and garden tools where your puppy cannot get to them and make sure they will not fall over if your puppy bumps into them.

❧ If you have a yard, consider adding a fence to keep your puppy in.

❧ Never leave them alone in a back yard, because even a fenced yard is little deterrent to a motivated English Springer Spaniel who has no fear of heights and is smart enough to figure out how to escape.

❧ Avoid using toxic chemical fertilizers, pesticides, or herbicides anywhere your puppy could be exposed – this includes toxic carpet and floor cleaning products.

Once you have puppy-proofed your home, the next step is to set up your puppy's area. You can choose a small room or use a puppy playpen to cordon off a section of a larger room. Place your puppy's crate and dog bed in the area as well as their food and water bowls and their toys. You will want to put your puppy in this area when you cannot actively watch him or her so they are less likely to get into trouble. While your puppy is very young, when you cannot closely watch them, you may want to confine him or her to their crate until they are housetrained.

Grooming Your Dog

Regular grooming is important for a happy and healthy dog, because it keeps them clean, and their skin moisturized and bug free, plus grooming time can alert you to any problems before they become more serious. Especially for longer-haired dogs, it will also be a good idea to commit to at least a weekly brushing or combing to remove debris and any tangled or matted hair.

 The English Springer Spaniel coat has long feathers that can quickly get tangled, which means extra time to brush or comb out this dog every few days.

Hair Brushing Technique

- Use a wire-pin brush or a soft bristle brush to brush out your dog's coat at least twice a week.

- Start at the base of the neck and work your way down the back and sides, always brushing in the direction of hair growth.

- Next, brush down each leg then have your dog roll over so you can brush out their underside. Don't forget the tail.

- If you happen to find a snag, work through it gently with your fingers, so you do not cause painful hair pulling that can hurt your dog.

- You can also use a comb to keep on top of tangles or mats, and the best comb is one that has rotating teeth, as this helps to prevent painful hair pulling.

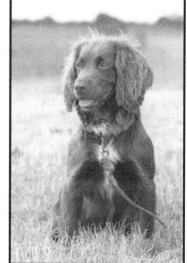

Depending upon whether you decide to fully groom your dog yourself, or will take him or her to the local doggy spa, you will require minimal equipment to keep the coat of your happy English Springer Spaniel looking his or her best. If you're just keeping on top of weekly brushing, all you will need is a soft bristle brush, pin brush or comb, and perhaps a flea comb (just in case). If you're planning to do all your dog's grooming yourself, see *"Grooming Equipment You Will Need"* on the next page.

Also, it will be very important to get this dog used to their grooming routine early on, because during their lifetime they will spend a lot of time at the grooming salon. Otherwise, every time your dog needs to be bathed, brushed and clipped will end up being a traumatic experience for both dog and human that can last for many years. Start them off right so you can both enjoy grooming time.

 I've been asked to groom dogs that have been kicked out of every grooming salon because their owners did not take the time to introduce the puppy to bath time, nail trimming and hair clipping procedures at a young age.

I can tell you from much personal experience that having to groom a writhing, screaming dog that is all teeth, because they are fighting the procedure, is hell on wheels, and the very worst case I ever encountered was with a dog weighing only 4 pounds (1.8 kg). Try going through this with an unwilling much larger English Springer Spaniel, and you will very soon be wishing your companion were a chia pet.

Grooming Equipment You Will Need

A standard arsenal of equipment for the DIY groomer that will help you keep your dog looking their best will include the following:

Bristle/Pin brush combination (pictured) – is the ideal tool for removing dirt and debris from the English Springer Spaniel's coat, while at the same time distributing natural oils to keep the coat looking healthy and shiny.

Sturdy Metal Comb – get one that has rotating teeth as this pulls the hair much less.

Slicker Brush – this has rows of metal teeth placed closely together and is a great tool for smoothing the coat.

Grooming Clipper (pictured) – this is an essential tool for anyone planning to learn how to groom their own dog's ever-growing coat.

There are electric ones and cord-free, rechargeable ones. Get a quality, professional grade clipper as these cut the hair much easier, are quieter and will last a long time. Rather than using snap-on plastic combs for different coat lengths (which are usually too flimsy for an English Springer Spaniel coat), I recommend spending the extra money to purchase the proper length metal blade attachment. Each electric clipper comes with a very short #1 blade attached. If you want to give this fur friend a puppy clip to make them more comfortable during the warmer winter months, you'll need a professional clipper.

 I find that a #4 blade is perfect for most coats, summer and winter, as it gives a good, smooth puppy cut when grooming in the direction of the hair growth that's just the right length. When you run against the growth of the hair, you can get a very short summer clip with this same blade.

Nail clippers (pictured) or a slow speed pet Dremel™ – will be tools you need to use every couple of weeks or more, depending on how quickly your dog's nails grow and what types of surfaces they may be walking on. The pet Dremel is perfect for smoothing the sharp edges that nail clippers leave, and if you are vigilant with regular use of the Dremel, you may never have to clip.

Flea comb (pictured) – hopefully you won't ever need one, however, as the name suggests, these combs are designed for the specific purpose of removing fleas from a dog's coat. Usually small in size for manoeuvring in tight spaces, they may be made of plastic or metal with the teeth of the comb placed very close together to trap hiding fleas.

Tick Twister (pictured) – hopefully your dog won't ever get a tick, but if they do, this is a simple device for painlessly, easily and quickly removing ticks that have imbedded themselves in your dog's skin.

Grooming Products You Will Need

Products you will need to invest in when bathing your dog yourself will include shampoos, conditioners, creams, lotions, sprays and powders.

Shampoos: NEVER make the mistake of using human shampoo or conditioner that has a pH balance of 5.5, for bathing your dog. Our canine companions have an almost neutral pH balance of 7.5, and any shampoo with a lower pH will be harmful to your dog, because it will strip the natural oils and be too harshly acidic for their coat and skin, which can create itchy skin problems and allow for a very unhappy dog.

Conditioners: taking the extra time to condition your dog's coat will not only make it look and feel better, it will also add additional benefits, including:

- Preventing the escape of natural oils and moisture

- Keeping the coat cleaner for a longer period of time

- Repairing a coat that has become dull, damaged or dry

- Restoring a soft, silky feel

- Helping the coat dry more quickly

❧ Protecting from the heat of the dryer and breakage of hair

The benefits of spending the extra two minutes to condition your dog's coat will be appreciated by both yourself and your dog that will have overall healthy, moisturized skin and a coat with a natural shine.

Bathing your dog:

❧ To bathe your dog, simply fill your bathtub with a few inches of lukewarm water and place your dog in it – you can put a bath mat or towel down to keep him or her from slipping.

❧ Then, use a cup or a hand sprayer to wet down your dog's coat and work a little bit of dog-friendly shampoo into a thick lather.

❧ Rinse the coat well until the coat is completely free of all of the shampoo suds, squeeze out the excess water with your hands and then towel your dog dry.

❧ Unless your dog gets dirty, you should only plan to bathe him or her once every 4 to 6 weeks because bathing too often can dry out your dog's skin and coat.

Oops, My Dog Has Fleas

You haven't been paying attention and now realize that your dog is suffering from an infestation of fleas. Now is the time to bathe them with shampoo containing pyrethrum (a botanical extract found in small, white daisies) or a shampoo containing citrus or tea tree oil.

Also, you can bathe and spray them with the non-toxic and highly effective CedarCide products, which can also be used to spray down their bedding and any carpets in the home, and will kill fleas (or other crawly creatures) on contact without harming anyone.

CedarCide is a company that makes 100% safe, organic products to control biting bugs on your furry friends without worrying about harmful chemicals that are not good for you, your children or your canine companions because it's safe to use on dog and human alike.

Simply spray it on and bugs of any sort that come into contact with the solution will be dead, while your dog's coat will be shiny and fresh smelling, like the inside of a cedar chest.

Nail Care

Many canine guardians neglect taking proper care of their dog's toenails, which can lead to many problems later in life, such as painful joints, back pain and difficulty walking, which will make for a very unhealthy and unhappy dog.

Purchase a good pair of medium-sized, scissor-type nail clippers with a safety stop and learn how to properly use them. If you don't, your dog's nails will soon be too long and the vein inside the nail will also grow too long and you will be unable to keep them as short as they should be.

Depending on the types of surfaces your English Springer Spaniel is walking on, you should plan to clip your dog's nails approximately every two weeks. When trimming the nails, be sure to only snip the tip, so you do not accidentally cut into the vein, which will be painful and will cause your dog to bleed.

Steps For Nail Clipping

- ❧ Hold your canine's paw firmly but gently.

- ❧ Trim the nail below the quick at a 45° angle, cutting small amounts at a time.

- ❧ Trim small slices until you reach the white inside the nail with a small black dot at the centre. If you can't see the dot yet, and all you are seeing is completely white, you can cut a bit more.

TIP *If your puppy has not had their "dew claws" removed (these are the claws that are on the side of the foot that never touch the ground), they still continue to grow. If you miss clipping these nails, they will soon grow into a circle that will be very difficult to clip and can even grow back into the dog's leg causing great pain.*

Styptic Powder: you will always want to avoid causing any pain when trimming your English Springer Spaniel's toenails, because you don't want to destroy their trust in you regularly performing this necessary task.

However, accidents do happen, therefore if you clip too short, and accidentally cut into the vein in the toenail, know that you will cause your dog pain, and that the toenail will bleed. Therefore, it is always a good idea to keep some styptic powder (often called *"Kwik Stop")* in your grooming kit.

Dip a moistened finger into the powder and apply it with pressure to the end of the bleeding nail, because this is the quickest way to stop a nail from bleeding in just a few seconds.

Some dogs prefer having their nails trimmed with a rotary "Dremel" type of device that grinds down the excess nail. There are several benefits inherent in using this tool for keeping your dog's nails trimmed, including: (a) it is easier to avoid cutting into the vein; (b) many dogs prefer it because there is no squeezing or clicking sound; (c) you can smoothly round the nails so there will be no sharp edges; and (d) when you use this tool every week, you can trim shorter and will never have to actually clip the nails.

TIP *Keep in mind that if you decide to trim your dog's nails this way, you* **MUST** *purchase a "doggy Dremel" made especially for this purpose (pictured), because using your shop Dremel will harm your dog's nails as it is too high speed and will burn* *the nails.*

Ear Care

Dogs can often suffer from painful ear infections, especially dogs like the English Springer Spaniel, that have fairly large, upright ears, because these ears can easily trap foreign objects.

Paying attention and keeping your dog's ears clean and dry will prevent this type of unhappy pain and suffering. If you notice your dog scratching at their ears, moaning, crying or constantly shaking their head, it's time for a trip to the vet's office. Make sure that you keep ear powders and cleaning solutions in your grooming kit, because with proper preventative care, you can help to prevent your dog from ever having to suffer from an irritating and painful ear infection.

Ear Powders: which can be purchased at any pet store, are designed to help keep your dog's ears dry while at the same time inhibiting the growth of bacteria that can lead to infections. Ear powders are also used when removing excess hair growth from inside a dog's ear canal, as the powder makes it easier to grip the hair.

Ear Cleaning Solutions: your local pet store will offer a wide variety of ear cleaning creams, drops, oils, rinses or wipes specially formulated for cleaning your English Springer Spaniel's ears.

In addition, there are many home remedies that will just as efficiently clean your dog's ears without the high price tag, including Witch Hazel (a 50:50 solution of Organic Apple Cider Vinegar and Purified Water) or a 50:50 solution of Hydrogen Peroxide and Purified Water.

Cleaning your dog's ears

- ❖ Lift your dog's ear, holding it between your thumb and forefinger to get a good look inside the ear.

🐾 Check for redness, discharge or bad smell. It is normal to see a small amount of light-coloured wax. If there is a very large amount, the ears are red, or there appears to be pus or a bad smell, this is a sign of a problem that will require immediate veterinary attention.

🐾 Gently wipe around the entrance of the ear canal with damp cotton wool, removing dirt or excess wax.

🐾 Insert the tip of the bottle into the ear canal making sure not to insert it too far, and then squeeze the bottle to release the ear cleaner.

🐾 Massage the base of the ear to help the cleaner pass inside the ear canal.

🐾 Wipe away any excess cleaner amount with damp cotton wool.

🐾 Repeat the same process for the other ear.

🐾 If your vet has prescribed ear drops, it's best to apply them straight after you've finished cleaning the ears. This will ensure that the medicine will enter the ear effectively and be absorbed without being blocked by excess wax.

Teeth Care

Another greatly overlooked area in your happy English Springer Spaniel's health is ensuring that their teeth are clean and properly looked after, so that they don't suffer from loose or broken teeth, and plaque build-up that leads to painful gum disease. You know how miserable a toothache can be – imagine your poor dog that cannot tell you how unhappy they are.

Many guardians use the excuse that *"my dog doesn't like it"* when they try to brush their dog's teeth.

Do NOT give up and overlook the fact that in order to keep the entire dog healthy, they <u>must</u> have healthy teeth and the only way to ensure this, is to commit to making the time to brush your dog's teeth every day or two.

Canine Toothpastes: are flavoured with beef or chicken in an attempt to appeal to the dog's taste buds, and some contain baking soda, which is the same mild abrasive found in many human pastes, and are designed to gently scrub the teeth.

Other types of canine toothpastes are formulated with enzymes that are designed to work chemically by breaking down tartar or plaque in the dog's mouth. While these pastes don't need to be washed off your dog's teeth and are safe for them to swallow, whether or not they remain on the dog's teeth long enough to do any good might be debatable.

Just as effective for killing germs, whitening and cleaning your dog's teeth, and much less expensive than fancy pastes, is old-fashioned hydrogen peroxide; you can also combine hydrogen peroxide (3% food grade), Aloe Vera juice (1:1) with a little bit of baking soda.

How can I brush my dog's teeth?

In the beginning, it is important to get your dog used to the toothpaste and to the whole brushing experience. Here is the technique I use:

- ❖ Check your dog's teeth and gums often to see what is normal so you can spot any issues or problems.

- ❖ During the first few days, hold your dog as you would normally when you are petting him or her.

- ❖ Gently stroke the outside of the cheeks with your finger for 1 or 2 minutes.

- After each session, reward your dog with praise and a treat they like. For the next few days, after your dog has become comfortable with this activity, place a small amount of toothpaste on your finger and let your dog try the flavour.

- Next, you should introduce your dog to a canine toothbrush or finger brush.

- Apply a pea-sized amount of toothpaste that has been specially formulated for dogs on the brush. Gently lift your dog's upper lip and place the brush against an upper tooth.

- With a slow circular motion, brush gently only that tooth and the adjoining gum line.

- Every following day gradually increase the number of teeth being brushed. Remember to go slowly, and do not continue beyond your dog's point of comfort.

- Build up to 30 seconds of brushing per side.

- The easiest way to do this is to go straight, pushing the brush gently from front to back along the gum line. Next, add in the gentle circular motion.

- You do not have to brush the inside of the teeth, as the tongue keeps that side relatively free of plaque.

- After each session reward your dog with a treat and lots of praise.

- Ideally, brushing should be done every day, but if you miss 1-2 days per week, that would not be a big concern.

 The easiest and most effective way to brush a dog's teeth is with an electric toothbrush (the rotary type) that does all the work for you. You can easily slowly introduce this method, just as you did with the manual brush, and once your dog gets used to the buzzing, all you have to do is hold the brush against their teeth.

Paw Care

If your dog runs over sharp barnacles on the beach, jogs with you on hard road surfaces, or over other rough terrain, this can cause cuts and scrapes and very rough surfaces on the paws. If you live in a hot climate, be aware that sidewalks, road surfaces and sandy beaches can get extremely hot for your dog's feet.

Paw Creams: depending upon activity levels and the types of surfaces our canine counterparts usually walk on, they may suffer from cracked or rough pads. You can restore resiliency and keep your dog's paws in healthy condition by regularly applying a cream or lotion to protect their paw pads that is especially formulated for dogs. A good time to do this is just after you've clipped their nails.

In a Nutshell

Learning about simple steps that will keep your English Springer Spaniel safe, and being aware of what's involved in keeping him or her properly groomed will go a long way toward helping them to live a long, happy and healthy life.

While for many people the concept of grooming a dog conjures up notions of brushes and bows, it is in fact a vital element to their overall health and wellbeing.

Whether you decide to hand strip when the undercoat is shedding or regularly puppy clip this dog (or hire someone to do it for you), clipping their nails and brushing their teeth is essential and will help you detect any underlying diseases or conditions early and will allow your beloved fur friend to feel better and live longer, healthier and happier.

Chapter 9: Are YOU the Ideal Happy English Springer Spaniel Guardian?

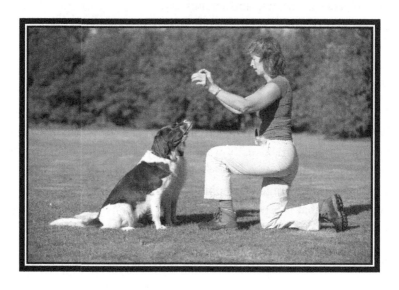

"A dog is the only thing on earth that loves you more than he loves himself."
— Josh Billings

If you have not chosen wisely when sharing your life with a canine companion, he or she will not be happy and neither will you, because you will be setting yourself, your family, your friends and your neighbours up for many years of stress, guilt and unhappiness.

It is vitally important that you take a good, hard look at your own energy level and lifestyle, ask yourself some serious questions that you honestly answer, and not scrimp on taking the time to do plenty of research about the breed of dog you may be considering.

Sharing your life with a canine friend should never be undertaken lightly, or on a whim or spur of the moment decision, or because you like the colour of a dog's coat or the sweet expression on their face.

Do You Have What It Takes?

Before you can learn how to become your dog's ideal guardian, you need to first have no doubt in your mind that you have the energy, commitment, time and skill level necessary to raise a happy dog. Once this is established in the affirmative, you then need to know how to choose the right breed of puppy or dog.

Choosing the <u>right</u> puppy for your family and your lifestyle is more important than you might imagine, and far too many people forget to consider how vital it is to choose a puppy or dog based on an honest assessment of compatibility with their own energy and lifestyle.

For instance, many humans choose a puppy (or older dog) for all the <u>wrong</u> reasons, including because:

- 🐾 they like what it looks like
- 🐾 the breed may currently be popular
- 🐾 they like that this dog's coat is beautiful
- 🐾 the breed appeared on TV or in a movie they enjoyed
- 🐾 their parents had the same kind of dog when they were a child
- 🐾 a friend or someone they admire has the same breed
- 🐾 they feel sorry for a homeless dog
- 🐾 a friend or family member can no longer keep their dog
- 🐾 the children are begging for a dog
- 🐾 someone was selling puppies on a street corner

While some of these above reasons can be honourable, the most important reasons for choosing to share your life with a particular canine companion has not been properly considered.

In order to make an intelligent choice that will bring happiness to everyone, you need to take a serious look at your life as it is today and also how you envision it to be during the next ten to fifteen years, and then ask yourself several very important questions, including:

Activity – Do I lead a highly active, medium or low-intensity life? For

"Can't take my dog?! But I don't even know HOW to run without my dog!"

instance, am I out jogging the streets every morning, hiking local mountains or riding my bicycle five miles to the local grocery store? Does my job keep me away from home, or does my leisure time activity keep me in front of the computer or on the couch watching movies?

Travel – Do I travel a lot for work or pleasure? If you do, perhaps you should choose a small dog that can travel with you in the plane cabin. Your loyal dog will be unhappy without you or you will have greatly increased expenses, because you will have to hire a dog sitter or leave them in a kennel.

Special Needs – do I have the extra finances required to keep an English Springer Spaniel well groomed? Am I able to keep this loyal dog at my side throughout most of every day?

Allergies – Do I prefer a very tidy house? Do I have allergies? This dog sheds their hair year round and much more when they blow their undercoat once or twice yearly. If you or a family member has allergies, the English Springer Spaniel may not be a good choice for allergy sufferers and neat freaks.

Time – Does my family take up all my spare time and are my children old enough to handle a puppy? A dog is like a child that never grows up and in order for them to be happy and well-behaved family members, they require a LOT of your daily time and attention.

Fitness – Am I physically fit and healthy enough to be out there walking and exercising a dog two to three times a day, every day, rain or shine, and much more during the puppy stage? Do I have the time to involve them in a canine sport or job? Remember that this dog needs at least 1-2 hours of vigorous activity every day.

Cost – Am I able to afford the extra food costs, trips to the grooming parlour, health insurance, licensing, appropriate clothing and the veterinarian expenses that are part of being a conscientious guardian?

Commitment – Is the decision to bring a puppy or dog into my life a family decision, or just because the children, who may quickly lose interest, have been begging for a dog?

Why? – What is the number one reason why I want a dog in my life?

Once you ask yourself these important questions and honestly answer them, you will have gained a much better understanding of whether or not you have what it takes to share your life with a dog, and perhaps the beginning insight of the type of puppy or dog that would be best suited for you and your family.

If you're too busy for a dog, or choose the wrong dog that is not compatible with you or your family's energy and lifestyle (or you don't really have the time, finances, patience, expertise and commitment necessary to properly socialize, train, exercise, feed, groom, raise and care for a canine companion), you will inevitably end up with an unhappy dog. This will lead to behavioral issues, which then will lead to a stressed family, angry neighbors, and in a best-case scenario, extra expenses to hire a professional to help you reverse unwanted behavioral problems.

Even worse, an incompatible choice can mean that you may end up contributing to the already overflowing crisis of yet another dog being abandoned at the local SPCA or kill shelter.

Once you have done all your homework, and absolutely determined that the loyal, super smart, agile and athletic English Springer Spaniel is the right dog for you (see next Section: The Ideal Guardian), rather than simply leaving it to chance, you need to choose the right puppy from the litter.

How to Choose Your English Springer Spaniel Puppy

Generally speaking, when choosing a puppy out of a litter, look for one that is friendly and outgoing, rather than one who is overly aggressive or fearful.

Visit the breeder and take note of a puppy's social skills when they are still with their littermates, because this will help you to choose the right puppy for your family. Puppies who demonstrate good social skills with their littermates are much more likely to develop into easy-going, happy adults who play well with other dogs.

In a social setting where all the puppies can be observed together, there are several important observations you can make, including:

Play – Notice which puppies are comfortable both on top and on the bottom when play fighting and wresting with their littermates, and which puppies seem to only like being on top. Puppies who don't mind being on the bottom or who appear to be fine with either position will usually play well with other dogs when they become adults.

Sharing – Observe which puppies try to keep the toys away from the other puppies and which puppies share. Those who want to hoard the toys and keep all other puppies away may be more aggressive with other dogs over food or treats, or in play where toys are involved as they become older.

Company – Notice which puppies seem to like the company of the other pups and which ones seem to be loners. Puppies who like the company of their littermates are more likely to be interested in the company of other dogs as they mature, rather than anti-social puppies.

Compassion – Observe the reaction of puppies that get yelped at when they bite or roughhouse with another puppy too hard. Puppies who ease up when another puppy yelps or cries are more likely to respond appropriately when they play too roughly as adults.

Sociability – Check to see if the puppy you are interested in is sociable with people, because if they will not come to you, or display fear of strangers, this may develop into a fear/aggression problem when they become adults.

Handling – Check if the puppy you are interested in is relaxed about being handled, because if they are not, they may become difficult or overly nervous around adults and children during daily interactions, during grooming or while visiting the veterinarian's office.

Is Your Happy Puppy Healthy?

While mental health is very important, you will also want to do all you can to determine if your chosen puppy is physically healthy.

First, ask to see veterinarian reports from the breeder to satisfy yourself that the puppy is as healthy as possible, and then once you make your decision to share your life with a particular puppy, and they are old enough to bring home, make an appointment with your own veterinarian for a complete examination.

However, before you take your new puppy home, there are general signs of good health to be aware of, including the following:

Body Fat – a healthy puppy will look round and well fed, with an obvious layer of fat over their rib cage.

Breathing – a healthy puppy will breathe quietly, without coughing, wheezing or sneezing.

Coat Condition – a healthy puppy will not be itchy and will have a soft coat with no dandruff, dullness, greasiness or bald spots.

Energy Level – a well-rested puppy will be alert and energetic.

Hearing – a healthy puppy should react if you clap your hands or snap your fingers behind their head.

Genitals – a healthy puppy will not have any sort of discharge visible in or around their genital or anal regions.

Mobility – a healthy puppy will walk and run normally without wobbling, limping or seeming to be weak, stiff or sore.

Vision – a healthy puppy will have bright, clear eyes without crust or discharge and they should notice if a ball is rolled past or a toy is tossed within their field of vision.

The Ideal Guardian Profile

Once you have established that you have what it takes to share your life with a dog (by considering the questions in the previous Section), you should consider the following tips to determine whether the English Springer Spaniel would be the right breed for you and your family.

The English Springer will be an excellent choice for moderate to high-energy individuals or families who live in a large home with a yard or on a property or hobby farm, and older children that understand how to respect a dog that has considerable mental and physical exercise needs. This dog could be a good companion for active senior adults who have the energy, time and mobility required to provide this athletic companion with the vigorous daily exercise and mental stimulation they need.

Keep in mind that while a well-socialized dog will usually be accepting and friendly toward both unknown dogs and humans; when not trained to heed their guardian's lead and not adequately socialized, this dog could become bossy, or nervous in unfamiliar situations, which can lead to unwanted aggression. Any dog that is babied too much can develop behavior problems. For instance, while the English Springer Spaniel is usually respectful toward everybody, it is possible for any canine to become snappish if they think leadership has defaulted to them.

The ideal guardian for the Happy English Springer Spaniel will be a person who understands the importance of firm rules and boundaries for their dog, who is retired or works at home, and enjoys several energetic daily walks plus off leash time to freely run, and some time for play or a canine sport. This guardian will also be aware of this dog's high stamina and strong desire to please, and that they may develop depression, frustration, a nervous disposition or separation anxiety (that leads to destructive behavior and escape attempts), if they are expected to spend long hours alone every day.

This ideal guardian will also understand the basics of socializing and firm, fair training, without raised voices, and may also enjoy teaching this companion tricks and/or a fun canine sport, and be willing to involve him or her in their own daily walking, biking, swimming, jogging or hiking routine.

As an example, this dog's guardian will be someone who works at home or is retired, and takes his or her dog out for a brisk 30-minute walk, so they can empty their bladder and bowels first thing every morning before breakfast, rain or shine, plus some off leash time where they can run freely chasing and retrieving a ball or socializing and playing with other dogs.

After returning home, everyone will have their breakfast and then (since you work at home or are retired) your dog can relax on the couch for a couple of hours while you work about the home. Before long it's noon and time to leash up your companion and head off for a longer walk. Depending on the weather, you may finish up at the lake or ocean side for a game of fetch in the water. If it's a hot day out, always carry water for your dog, and don't let them play too long.

Back home for a midday dental snack for your dog and lunch for you, while you take time (depending on this dog's age) to teach basic commands, play a short game in the back yard, maybe teach some tricks, or head off to the local Agility or Flyball course.

Now it's about 4:00 pm and again it's time to get you and your dog outside for a 30-minute walk around the block, or perhaps hitch them up to a Springer bicycle jogger and let them jog beside your bicycle.

Then if it's not too hot or too cold out, perhaps another short stop at the park for socializing and running free with other dogs.

 Keep in mind that if you live where the winters are harsh and you have access to a treadmill, this dog can quickly be taught to exercise indoors alongside you on a treadmill.

Back home and time to prepare dinner for both dog and human, then after dinner (again depending on the age of your dog) perhaps a few more minutes of basic command and/or trick training before you head off to the local dog park for a game of Frisbee.

Now it's getting to be later evening and before bed you need to put your dog on leash and take them outside for a few minutes so they can drain out their bladder before bed.

Everyone now in his or her respective beds as both human and dog have a rejuvenating sleep before the start of the next day when you do this (or something similar) all over again.

Of course, this is just one scenario that would be excellent for the Happy English Springer Spaniel, and with a little imagination on your part, there are many others that would fit the bill quite nicely.

Also, don't forget to check out your local weekend canine sporting facilities, and take the time to get you and your dog involved, because your weekend would be well spent teaching this dog how to run an Agility course, or perhaps participate in Advanced Obedience or even a Barn Hunt competition.

In a Nutshell

While learning how to choose the right puppy is important, even more important is your ability to ask and honestly answer the questions outlined in this Chapter that will help you to understand if you truly are a good fit for being the ideal guardian for this canine Einstein, who will be your devoted and loving companion for many years.

Remember that if you don't really have the time, commitment and knowledge necessary to properly socialize, train and raise this versatile and energetic companion (that includes daily mental and physical exercise), you will inevitably end up with an unhappy dog. This will lead to health and behavioral issues, which then will lead to a stressed dog, a stressed family, possibly angry neighbors, and extra expenses to hire a professional to help you reverse unwanted behavioral problems, which is, of course, only possible if YOU are willing to make the necessary changes in your life.

Chapter 10: Humans Make a LOT of Stupid Mistakes

*"Heaven goes by favor. If it went by merit,
you would stay out and your dog would go in."*
— Mark Twain

Far too often we humans don't even realize we are the cause of creating behavioral problems in our canine companions, and when we're not aware and paying attention, we may be causing a lot of issues that can actually be entirely avoided.

Besides the more obvious problems that can arise with a dog that is bred for tracking, hunting, search and rescue or detection work and can become an unhappy member of your family when not raised properly and engaged in a working capacity, there are many other situations or unwanted outcomes that may arise that can be avoided.

For instance, there are many "mistakes" you can inadvertently make that can lead to plenty of troubles later in life, such as:

☙ not taking the time to properly socialize

- not desensitizing your dog to loud noises

- falling prey to those staring eyes that they know how to work to their own advantage

- feeding too much

- not exercising enough

- not finding ways to mentally challenge

- accidentally rewarding your dog at the wrong time

- allowing your dog to be the boss

- not being a strong enough leader for the dog you choose

- not having the knowledge you need to properly raise a dog

- not being aware of a particular breed's special needs

- not taking the time to teach basic rules and boundaries

- not being honest about your own energy level

- not being honest about how much time you can devote to a dog

All of these and more can inadvertently create unhappiness and unwanted behaviors that lead to health issues that could have been entirely avoided.

As well, not being aware of the adolescent craziness time in a young dog's life and how to get through it, and many other less obvious mistakes, such as choosing the wrong collar or leash, allowing your dog to sleep in your bed, or free feeding can all result in the creation of problems.

While we humans may be well meaning, besides the obvious disasters that we can create when we don't properly train or socialize our canine friends, we can inadvertently make a lot of stupid mistakes when raising our canine companions that will cause our fur friends to needlessly suffer.

Let's begin with the more obvious *"Preventing Socialization Behavioral Issues"* that can lead to problems later in life, and proceed further into areas of *"Accidental Rewards"* that may not be so obvious, then touch upon *"Basic Rules and Boundaries"* and *"Adolescent Craziness",* and finish this chapter with *"Less Obvious Stupid Human Mistakes".*

Preventing Socialization Behavioral Issues

In order to prevent behavioral issues you first need to be aware of how easy it is to inadvertently create them yourself.

Much of how your chosen dog learns to behave will depend entirely upon you, how extensively they were socialized as a puppy and how much they are continually being socialized throughout their life.

Without proper socialization, even the most naturally polite dog can become neurotic, overly bossy, nervous, unsociable, and learn to act out aggressively toward unknown dogs, smaller animals or people. This is a situation that can get any dog labelled nasty or even dangerous should they act out aggressively for any reason.

Many people don't realize how important it is to properly and continually socialize their dogs in several different areas.

 Without proper socialization, many behavioral problems could become a daily occurrence.

Never make the mistake of thinking that you only need to socialize your puppy during the first few months of their life and that they will then be fine for the rest of their life, because all dogs, including the English Springer Spaniel, require constant socializing.

As well, once they reach adolescence, their personality can really begin to assert itself, and this is when, without constant and vigilant daily socializing and training, any nervous, aggressive or anti-social tendencies may begin to erupt.

Generally speaking, the majority of an adult dog's habits and behavioral traits will be formed between the ages of birth and one year of age. While it is even more important to introduce puppies to a wide variety of sights, sounds, smells and situations during the most formative period in their young life, which is usually their first 16 weeks, all dogs, no matter their age, need to be exposed to different people, dogs, animals, places and unusual sights and sounds throughout their entire adult life.

Socializing With Unknown Dogs

Any dog, despite their natural personality, that is not regularly socialized may become shy, nervous, afraid, suspicious or overly bossy around unfamiliar or unusual dogs, animals, people or circumstances, which could lead to nervous or fearful behavior, which can then lead to unacceptable fear or dominance aggression.

Daily on-leash dog walks are great opportunities for your dog to see and possibly meet other dogs and different people, as well as practice proper behavior when out and about.

Remember to take it slowly and never put your fur friend in a situation where he or she feels uncomfortable or feels forced into being around other canines they may be uncomfortable with. Your dog should always be given the option to walk away, with lots of space.

When socializing a young puppy, remember to introduce him or her first to the *more calm and friendlier* of dogs, because introducing your small pup to a dog that may be overly boisterous or not so friendly with other dogs may result in a negative experience.

Negative experiences at a young age may later result in a fear of other dogs. I would suggest finding a local puppy class with around 8-10 other puppies, so that you can carefully supervise socializing and guided play.

Socializing With Unknown People

Proper socialization also means taking your puppy (or dog) everywhere with you and introducing them to many different people of all ages, sizes and ethnicities, so they will learn what is normal and acceptable in their daily life.

 DO NOT get into the habit of always carrying a puppy or smaller dog. They need to walk on their own feet so that they don't develop unwanted behavior problems, such as "armpit alligator" tendencies (snapping when someone stops to say hello) that can result from being in an elevated position where they feel they are in charge and must protect their human.

 Also important, will be getting your puppy or dog used to the noise and unpredictable actions of young children. You will want to closely supervise play, so that children are not accidentally being too rough or screaming in high-pitched voices, because this can be very frightening for a sensitive young puppy or dog that is unfamiliar with children.

Be especially careful when introducing your puppy to young children who may accidentally hurt your puppy, because you don't want your dog to become fearful of children as this could lead to aggression issues later on in life. While this puppy is usually patient and gentle with children, any dog that is pushed too far may feel the need to protect his or herself from a child that is invading their space or treating them roughly.

Environmental Socialization

It can be a BIG mistake not to take the time to introduce your English Springer Spaniel puppy to a wide variety of different environments, because when they are not comfortable with different sights, smells and sounds, this could cause them (and you) stress and trauma later in their adult life.

Be creative and take your puppy everywhere you can imagine when they are young, so that no matter where they travel, whether strolling along a noisy city sidewalk or beside a peaceful shoreline, they will be equally comfortable. Also, don't forget to train this dog to like travelling inside their kennel when driving anywhere.

Do not make the mistake of only taking your puppy into areas where you live and will frequently travel, because they need to also be comfortable visiting areas you might not often visit, such as noisy construction sites, airports or a shopping area across town.

Your puppy needs to see all sorts of sights, sounds and situations so that they will not become fearful, should they need to travel with you outside of their immediate neighbourhood.

Your dog will take their cues from you, which means that when you are calm and in control of every situation, they will learn to be the same because they will trust and calmly follow your lead.

For instance, take them to a noisy construction site, to the airport where they can watch people and hear planes landing and taking off, to a local park where they can see a baseball game, for a stroll beside a schoolyard at recess time when noisy children are out playing, or to the local zoo or farm and let them get a close up look at horses, pigs and ducks. Use your imagination.

 Again, never think that socialization is something that only takes place when your dog is a young puppy, as proper socialization is on-going for your dog's entire life.

Fear of Loud Noises

Many dogs can show extreme fear of loud noises, such as fireworks, sirens, thunderstorms or home security alarms. We humans need to learn how to either prevent this trauma in the first place or learn how to appropriately respond to a dog that is afraid of loud noises.

When you take the time to desensitize your dog to these types of noises when they are very young, it will be much easier on them during stormy weather, holidays such as Halloween or New Year's, when fireworks are often a part of the festivities, when an ambulance or fire truck roars past with sirens wailing, or when your fire or security alarm is activated.

REMEMBER: Loud, piercing noises will be very painful for a dog's sensitive ears, so use your hands to protect their ears if you're out walking when a vehicle with a blaring siren is roaring past.

Desensitization Devices: there are several ways you can help to desensitize your dog, so that they are not fearful of high-pitched alarms, and loud, popping noises, including the following:

CDs: you can purchase CD's that are a collection of unusual sounds, such as vacuums or hoovers, airplanes, sirens, smoke alarms, fireworks, people clapping hands, screaming children, and more (or you can easily make your own), that you can play while working in your kitchen or relaxing in your living room or lounge.

When you play these sounds and pretend that everything is normal, the next time your puppy or dog hears these types of sounds elsewhere, they will not become upset or agitated because they have learned to ignore them.

Bubble Wrap: is also another simple way to desensitize a dog that is fearful of unexpected popping sounds. Show them the bubble wrap, pop a few of the cells and if they do not run away, give them a treat. You can start with the bubble wrap that has small, quieter cells, and then graduate them to the larger celled (louder) bubble wrap. You can also take things even farther by blowing up some small paper bags or balloons and loudly popping them in front of your dog, or taking them to the rifle range.

Thunder Shirts: some dogs will respond well to wearing a *"Thunder Shirt"*, which is specifically designed to alleviate anxiety or trauma associated with loud rumbling, popping or banging noises. The idea behind the design of the Thunder Shirt is that the gentle pressure it creates is similar to a hug that, for some dogs, has a calming effect.

Relaxation Collars: there are basically two types of collars designed to help relax or calm an upset puppy or dog. One uses scent or calming pheromones, while the other uses species-specific music at appropriate decibel levels to calm a fearful or stressed dog.

TV or Radio: sometimes all that is required to calm a dog that is stressed by loud noises is to play your inside TV or Radio station with the sounds of relaxing music, louder than you might normally, to help disguise the exterior noise of fireworks or thunder.

Always be aware that some dogs literally lose their minds and do things that make no logical sense when they hear the loud popping or screeching noises of fireworks and various alarms and start trembling, running or trying to hide and you cannot communicate with them at all.

Make certain that your dog cannot harm itself trying to escape from these types of noises, and if possible, calmly hold them until they begin to relax.

For instance, my dog, Boris, used to try and escape through the drain in the bathtub (go figure), because loud popping noises literally caused him to lose his mind.

Make sure that YOU are acting appropriately yourself, by not panicking or having weak, *"feeling sorry"* or *"angry and frustrated"* energy around an upset dog, because this will only make matters worse.

When the person who is supposed to be your dog's support system is also feeling weak or acting unstable, your dog will have nowhere to turn. Instead, support them by pretending that nothing is wrong and if you must talk to them, do so in a calm, yet assertive voice.

Never underestimate the importance of taking the time to continually (not just when they are puppies) socialize and desensitize your dog to all manner of sounds. Doing so will help curb their tendency to sound off at every little noise, which will make everyone happier in the future, while teaching them to be a calm and well-balanced member of your family in every situation.

Accidental Rewards

Many times, we humans are guilty of accidentally rewarding our puppies and dogs for engaging in types of behavior we are not happy with, and the following are some of the more obvious things we may be doing that are inadvertently rewarding, and thus encouraging, an unwanted behavior.

Aggression Rewards

Many people unknowingly get into the habit of accidentally rewarding their puppies or dogs for displaying nervousness, fear, barking, growling or lunging at another dog or person by picking them up, talking soothingly, or offering them a treat. I see this happen all too often.

For instance, many people simply pick up their dog when he or she is acting in an unacceptable manner. Do NOT get into this bad habit.

Should you accidentally reward your dog by picking them up when they are displaying any sort of unbalanced energy, you will be teaching them to continue with this type of unwanted behavior and you'll be picking them up forever.

As well, picking up a small dog or puppy when they are growling, barking or acting out inappropriately, again rewards them and places them in a top dog position where they literally have just gained the higher ground.

A dog in the *"top dog"* position feels more confident and, depending on your energy, will usually then become more dominant than the person or dog they may have just growled at when they were at *"ground level"*.

Rather than accidentally rewarding your English Springer Spaniel for displaying unwanted behavior, the correct action to take in such a situation is to keep them on the ground, and gently correct your puppy or dog with firm yet calm energy (that is just a little stronger than the energy your dog is displaying) by distracting them with a firm *"No!"* and a quick sideways snap of the leash to get their attention back on you. This will "tell" your dog that they must let you deal with whatever situation has caused them to react badly.

If you allow a fearful, nervous, shy or bossy dog to deal with situations that unnerve them and cause them to bellow loudly or act out aggressively when they encounter unfamiliar circumstances, you will have created a problem that could escalate into something very serious.

The same is true of situations where a young puppy may feel the need to protect itself from a larger or older dog that may come charging in for a sniff or is acting confrontational. It's the human guardian's responsibility to protect their puppy or dog, so that they do not feel that they must react with fear or aggression in order to protect his or herself or the human at the other end of the leash.

No matter the age or size of your puppy or dog, allowing them to display aggression, loud barking or any sort of unwanted behavior toward another dog, animal or person is NEVER a laughing matter and this type of behavior must be immediately curtailed.

Excitement Rewards

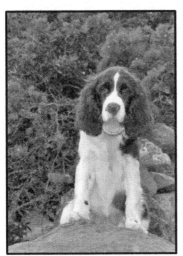

It's important to recognize that attention paid to an overly excited or out-of-control puppy or dog, even negative attention, is likely going to be rewarding for your fur friend. If your dog is not receiving enough of your attention, they will quickly learn to do whatever it takes to get the attention they desire.

Bottom line, when you engage with an out-of-control puppy or dog, you end up actually rewarding them for acting out in an unstable manner, and encouraging them to continue with more overly exuberant behavior you might not be very pleased about.

Be careful that you're not teaching your dog to act out with crazy energy every time they see you.

For instance, chasing after a puppy when they have taken something they are not supposed to have, picking them up when they're barking or showing aggression, pushing them off when they jump on you or other people, or yelling when they refuse to come when called, are all forms of negative attention that can actually be rewarding and encourage more of the same unwanted behavior.

Instead, remain calm and assertive and be consistent with your training, so that your dog learns how to control their energy and play quietly and appropriately without jumping on everyone or engaging in growling, barking or mouthy behavior.

Interaction Rewards

If your English Springer Spaniel displays excited energy simply from being petted by you, or anyone else, you will need to teach yourself, your family and your friends to ignore your fur friend until he or she calms down. Otherwise, you will be inadvertently teaching your canine companion that the touch of humans means excitement, and this behavioral problem will continue to escalate.

For instance, when you continue to engage with your overly excited puppy or dog, you are actually rewarding them for out-of-control behavior and literally teaching them that when they see humans, you want them to display excited energy.

Too many people encourage their dog to be nuts, for instance, when they return home and greet their dog in a highly excited state. While it's nice to know that your dog is happy to see you, when you forget about being your dog's calm pack leader just a few times, this may be enough to send your smart dog the message that they can no longer rely upon you to be their calm leader, and that seeing humans means they must now display out-of-control excitement.

Instead, when you come home, greet your dog calmly and quietly, and if they are at all excited, do NOT touch or talk to them until they calm down. Otherwise, your dog will soon learn that humans are a source of excitement, and long, consistently vigilant work on your part (with help from your friends and family) will be the only way to reverse this unwanted behavior.

Another thing to keep in mind is that children are often a source of high energy and excitement that can cause a puppy or dog to quickly become extremely wound up.

If you don't want to create an on-going behavioral problem, that could accidentally get someone injured, you will need to be very vigilant about NOT permitting young children to engage with an excited puppy or dog.

Important Basic Rules and Boundaries

You can prevent many future behavioral problems when you take the time to ensure that your chosen dog learns basic rules and boundaries. All that's necessary for effectively teaching your puppy (or dog) these basics is a calm, consistent and firm approach, combined with your endless patience.

Basic rules and boundaries would include things such as:

- 🐾 no barking at every little noise
- 🐾 no dogs allowed in the kitchen when preparing food
- 🐾 no begging at the human's dinner table

- 🐾 humans through the door first

- 🐾 no sleeping in the human bed

- 🐾 no raiding the garbage can

- 🐾 no jumping up on tables or counters

- 🐾 no jumping on humans

- 🐾 no helping yourself to "tootsie rolls" from the cat's litter box

- 🐾 no chasing the neighbor's cat

Many puppies are ready to begin basic training at about 10 to 12 weeks of age, and some will be ready at 8 weeks. However, be careful not to overdo it when they are less than four months of age, as their attention span may be short.

With younger puppies, make your training sessions no more than 5 or 10 minutes, positive and pleasant with plenty of praise and/or treats, so that your puppy will be looking forward to their next session.

Also, begin to introduce hand signals that go along with the verbal commands so that once they learn both, you can remove the verbal commands in favor of just hand signals.

When you teach a dog hand signals, they will become much more attentive because they must look at you to see what you require them to do.

Consistently teach your puppy or dog the *All Important Three*, which are the "Come", "Sit" and "Stay" commands (more about this in Chapter 12: Training Basics For a Happy English Springer Spaniel), and use them every day in every opportunity to help your young dog progress through their unpredictable adolescent period.

Adolescent Craziness

Too often, we humans become impatient and frustrated and give up on our dogs when they transition from being the cute, cuddly and mostly obedient little puppy they once were and become all kinds of craziness.

Instead of riding the adolescent storm, it is often during this confusing and trying adolescent stage of a dog's life that they end up behind bars when the humans who promised to love and protect them, abandon their once happy fur friend at the local SPCA or rescue facility.

With consistency, understanding, the right information, and endless patience and perseverance, you and your fur friend can emerge out the other side of this adolescent period with a much stronger bond.

Firstly, you need to know that not all dogs go through an intensely crazy adolescent period. Secondly, when you remain consistent with your socializing and training during this time, you can live through puppy adolescence and come out the other side a much more knowledgeable and patient guardian.

Remember, you've already lived through potty training, teething, socializing and basic rules and boundaries with your young dog, and you need to feel proud of all your accomplishments and the leaps and bounds you and your puppy have accomplished together over the last several months.

If your adolescent dog is now beginning to act out and push your buttons, rather than giving up on them, it's time to remain calm, consistent and <u>persistent,</u> and re-visit basic rules and boundaries, while keeping in mind that you will eventually be able to enjoy the happy rewards that all those months of diligent puppy training have brought to your relationship.

During adolescence, you may experience several changes in your dog's personality that you're not exactly pleased about. For instance, your young spaniel may:

- no longer be as friendly with strangers

- start to be possessive of their human

- start to bark at unknown people and dogs

- start to show their stubborn side

- ignore you when called

- appear to have suddenly gone deaf

- ignore the basic commands they've already learned

- start to relieve themselves inside again

- bark or cry when left alone

- begin to mark territory

- try to escape the back yard

Welcome to the world of canine adolescence, where it appears that all your previous work was for naught and your puppy has turned into some sort of monster.

DON'T PANIC, because every dog is different and your dog's adolescent period may go by without notice. However, being prepared for the worst will help you ride any impending storm and get you both safely out the other side where you can enjoy an even closer relationship than you previously had.

The adolescent phase may be very subtle for your puppy. On the other hand, it may be so dramatic that frustration with your fur friend is becoming a daily occurrence and you're questioning whether you made the right choice.

If frustration is getting the upper hand, rather than letting it get worse, consider the benefits of hiring a professional, who can provide insight and valuable assistance to help you through this stage of your puppy's development.

<u>Less Obvious Stupid Human Mistakes</u>

There are many less obvious mistakes we humans can inadvertently make with our dogs that can also lead to behavioral problems later in life, some of which include:

Sleeping in Your Bed: many people make the mistake of allowing an adorable crying puppy to sleep with them in their bed. While this may help to calm and comfort a new puppy, it will set a dangerous precedent that can result in behavioral problems later in their life, plus a sleeping human body could easily crush a small puppy.

As much as it may pull on your heart strings to hear your new puppy crying the first couple of nights in their kennel, a little tough love at the beginning will keep them safe while helping them to learn to both love <u>and</u> respect you as their leader.

FACT *Be aware that it's perfectly fine and natural for your puppy or dog to sleep in the same room with you. After all, they are part of your "pack" and need to be near. Just make sure that you don't let him or her take over YOUR bed.*

Picking Them Up at the Wrong Time: never pick your puppy up if they display nervousness, fear or aggression (such as growling) toward an object, person or other pet, because this will be rewarding them for unbalanced behavior.

Instead, your puppy needs to be gently corrected by you, with firm and calm energy, so that they learn not to react with fear or aggression.

Armpit Alligators: when your dog is a small puppy, be aware that many guardians get into the bad habit of carrying a small dog or puppy far too much.

Remember that they need to be on the ground and walking on their own, so that they do not become overly confident. A dog that is carried by their guardian is literally being placed in the *"top dog"* position.

Be aware that humans who constantly carry small dogs or puppies, rather than allowing them to walk on their own, can often inadvertently create what I refer to as an *"armpit alligator"* situation. This is where you see someone carrying a cute little dog and you stop to say hello, only to be greeted by snapping jaws and sharp teeth.

Even dogs that are usually polite (like the English Springer Spaniel) and not naturally wary or suspicious of strangers can learn to become intolerant if they don't receive adequate socialization, which means that it is always possible to allow them to become protective or possessive of *"their"* humans.

Playing Too Hard or Too Long: many humans play too hard or allow their children to play too long or too roughly with their puppy. You need to remember that your young puppy tires very easily and especially during the critical growing phases of their young life, they need their rest.

Hand Play: always discourage your puppy from chewing or biting your hands, or any part of your body for that matter, and dissuade this little herding from nipping at heels.

Do NOT get into the habit of playing the *"hand"* game, where you rough up your puppy and slide them across the floor with your hands, because this will teach them that your hands are playthings and you will have to work long and hard to break this bad habit.

PERSONAL EXPERIENCE: When my puppy came home with me at 10-weeks of age, the breeder had already been playing the hand game and it took me a very long time to teach my Boris that biting human hands was not acceptable behavior. Interestingly, when he sees people that he has not seen for years, that he used to know when he was a young puppy, this old habit often re-surfaces for a short while.

When your puppy is teething, they will naturally want to chew on everything within reach, and this will include you. As cute as you might think it is, this is not an acceptable behavior and you need to gently, but firmly, discourage the habit.

A light flick with a finger on the end of your puppy's nose, combined with a firm "NO" and removing the enticing fingers by making a fist when they are trying to bite those human fingers, will discourage them from this activity.

Not Getting Used to Grooming: not taking the time to get your dog used to a regular grooming routine, including bathing, brushing, toenail clipping and teeth brushing, can lead to a lifetime of trauma for both human and dog every time these procedures must be performed.

reminder *Set aside several minutes each day or two for your grooming routine.*

NOTE: get your puppy used to being up high on a table or countertop when you are grooming them. This way, when it comes time for a full grooming session or a visit to the vet's office, where they will be placed on an examination table, they will not be stressed because this will already be a familiar situation.

Free Feeding: means to keep food in your puppy's bowl 24/7, so that they can eat any time of the day or night, whenever they feel like it.

While free feeding a young puppy can be a good idea (especially with very small dogs), until they are about four or five months old, many guardians often get into the bad habit of allowing their adult dogs to continue to eat food any time they want, by leaving food out 24/7.

The English Springer Spaniel is usually quite food motivated, which means if there is food out they will probably eat it. However, while every dog is different, you don't want to get into the habit of leaving food out 24/7 because (a) they no longer associate you being in control of the food, and (b) if your particular dog gets used to eating too much, they will quickly gain weight and become obese, which can lead to health issues that may shorten their life.

Getting into a free feeding habit can be a serious mistake, as your dog is not a cat, and needs to know that you are absolutely in control of their food.

Treating Them Like Children: do not get into the bad habit of treating your dog like a small, furry human; even though they may try their best to please you and their doggy smarts could help them to succeed in most instances, not honoring them for the amazing dog they are will only cause them confusion that could lead to behavioral problems.

 Remember that the one thing your dog is the absolute BEST at, is Being a Dog.

A well-balanced dog thrives on rules and boundaries, and when they understand that there is no question that you are their leader and they are your follower, they can relax and live a contented, happy and stress-free life.

Distraction and Replacement: when your puppy tries to chew on your hand, foot, clothing, or anything else that is not fair game, you need to firmly and calmly tell them "No", and then distract them by replacing what they are not supposed to be chewing with something they <u>are</u> permitted to chew, such as an appropriate toy.

Make sure that you happily praise them every time they choose the toy to chew on. If your puppy persists in chewing on you, remove yourself from the equation by getting up and walking away. If they are really persistent, put them inside their kennel with a favorite chew toy until they calm down.

Always praise your puppy when they stop inappropriate behavior or replace inappropriate behavior with something that is acceptable to you, so that they begin to understand what they can and cannot do.

<u>Flat Collar Nightmares</u>

Many humans simply don't realize how important it is to choose the "right" kind of collar for their canine companion. Add this to the fact that there is an ever-increasing array of tempting colors and styles to choose from and it's very easy to get distracted and forget about choosing what you <u>really</u> need for your dog.

What you really need in a collar is one that will also keep your dog safe and secure. While the flat collar may be fine for a calm dog that never pulls, leaps about or suddenly tries to do an about face and take off running in a different direction to chase that teasing squirrel or taunting cat, this is not a very safe reality.

TIP *While you will choose what you will for your dog, after 40 some years of working with dogs and experiencing possibly every type of terrifying, unexpected disaster while out walking a dog, the ONLY collar I feel absolutely confident using (because I know that the dog I'm in control of cannot wiggle out of it), is the "Martingale" collar.*

Flat collars, unless you have them cinched up so tight that you're almost cutting off your dog's air supply, can be fairly easy for most dogs to get out of.

All dogs are amazing athletes, and even though you may have a firm grip on that leash, they can back away from you, wiggle, twist and contort themselves in a quick instant, flip their head and the collar is off – bye, bye doggy!

The Martingale Collar

There are several reasons why the Martingale dog collar **(see photo below)** is far superior to a flat collar:

- 🐾 comfortable for your dog to wear all day long

- 🐾 safe because your dog cannot wiggle out of it

- 🐾 best training collar

The Martingale collar looks much the same as a flat collar, with one very important difference – there is a triangular piece of chain in the middle of it. This chain is attached to the collar with two rings, with a third ring in the middle of the chain, which is where you attach your leash.

When there is no tension on the collar (from them pulling on the leash), the collar hangs loose and comfortable. However, when there IS tension on the collar, that little piece of chain tightens so that your dog cannot get out of their collar.

PERSONAL EXPERIENCE: My dog (despite his short nose) has been wearing the same Martingale "training" collar for almost 15 years and will continue to do so, because this collar conveys important messages between my dog and myself.

That little piece of triangular chain makes a slight noise when you sharply tug or jiggle it, and this sends a message to your dog that you want their attention on you. It's simply the best collar for teaching your dog to walk calmly by your side and to remind them that YOU are in charge.

When buying a Martingale collar for your English Springer Spaniel, take him or her with you because it needs to be the correct size to fit over the widest part of their head. Then, once you've got the right size for your dog, you need to pay strict attention to the <u>correct way to adjust</u> the collar for maximum effect and safety.

Adjusting the Martingale Collar: once you've placed the collar over your dog's head, it's important that you properly adjust it. You need to adjust the length so that when you attach the leash to the outside ring and pull it tight, when the two inside rings come together, there is still a gap between these two rings of approximately two human finger widths. You never want the two inside rings to touch.

You can now enjoy comfortable and safe walks with your Happy English Springer Spaniel companion.

Flexi-Leash Fiasco

Personally, flexi, retractable or extendable dog leashes **(see photo below)** are high on my list of pet peeves for several important reasons, including that they:

- 🐾 are dangerous for human and dog alike

- 🐾 allow the dog to be in the wrong walking position

- 🐾 allow the humans to forget their responsibilities

- 🐾 are heavy, clumsy and difficult to securely grip

- 🐾 are an excuse for not properly training your dog

- 🐾 can accidentally break

While many people believe that a retractable leash is a good way to allow their dogs more freedom to roam while still keeping them securely attached, the above reasons highlight why these leashes can be a very bad idea. See below for more details.

Injury to human and dog: these leashes are usually spring-loaded, many feet long (usually 26 feet or 7.9 meters), and thin cords wound up inside a cumbersome plastic compartment with a handle and a button to control how much of the leash is extended.

As you can imagine, it's far more difficult to control a dog that is roaming about 20 or more feet away from you, than it would be if they were attached to a standard 4 to 6 foot leash and walking at your side.

If your dog gets used to having a 20-foot (6 meter) or more leeway, they will be busy sniffing interesting scents, and can quickly run out into traffic, be surprised by another dog rushing in, or get tangled up with a person and a dog, which can cause both injury to the dogs and people, or may cause a fight between the two dogs.

These leashes are also serious tripping hazards that can cause many injuries.

MEMORY LANE: The daughter of one of my dog whispering clients broke her toe as a result of tripping over a flexi-leash, I have suffered painful "rope" burns several times, and once was hit in the head (ouch!) with the hard and heavy plastic handle as it snapped back when the person holding it lost their grip and dropped it.

In addition, every flexi or retractable leash is equipped with a brake to stop the unwinding of the cord at various lengths. If your dog is running and all of a sudden comes to the end of their freedom, unless you drop the handle, they will be forced to come to a very abrupt stop that can injure a dog's neck or spine.

Incorrect Walking Position: the ONLY place your dog should ever be when you're out walking is beside you, and when you allow them to freely roam 20 or more feet from wherever you are, besides being lax about teaching your dog the correct walking position, you are *"telling"* them that you are no longer in charge. A dog that believes they are in charge can get you BOTH into a lot of trouble.

Forgetting Your Human Responsibilities: when you're out walking with your puppy or dog, as their leader, you are responsible for everything they do, including picking up after them. A retractable leash allows your dog to literally be out of your sight. While you're busy chatting with a neighbor or checking your phone messages, you may not be aware of what sort of *"message"* your dog may be depositing in the neighbor's yard.

You can be fined for not picking up after your dog, not to mention gaining yourself a bad reputation from your neighbors or other more responsible dog walkers.

Difficult to Securely Grip: the flexi leash has a large, cumbersome handle that is quite slippery and difficult to securely hold onto. If your companion suddenly lunges or changes direction, the chances of you losing your grip are quite high, and when that happens, the consequences can be dangerously grave.

Once dropped, your dog is now dragging a bouncing, loudly clattering handle, which can be very noisy on a sidewalk or hard surface.

MEMORY LANE: This very thing has happened to me in a busy, high traffic area, when walking someone else's dog. While I was lucky and managed to get him safely back, I can tell you from first-hand experience that this is a highly stressful and frightening situation I would not want to wish on anyone.

Unless your dog has been trained to remain calmly sitting while rifles are fired near their head, this flexi leash that seems to be chasing them can be a very scary experience that will cause most dogs to run.

When your dog is scared, they will run even faster, while you run after them adding to the chaos with your panic-stricken screams to stop before they get killed trying to cross a busy intersection. Not a good scene.

Poor Training: while many might believe they are giving their dog more freedom by using a retractable leash, they are actually missing out on properly training their dog to heel beside them and to respond appropriately to the all-important "come" or "recall" command.

The very nature of a flexi leash is such that the dog is often out in front of the person who is supposed to be in charge, and always *"pulling"*, which to an approaching dog can look like an aggressive stance, resulting in the other dog thinking he or she must retaliate with a defensive stance. All of this, as you can imagine, has the potential to result in a scuffle between dogs and humans.

Accidental Breakage: there is a great deal of wear on a small diameter cord that is constantly unwinding and rewinding and you may not notice a worn area until it actually breaks. Then, you've got a potential runaway dog disaster to hopefully recover from, before the dog gets severely injured, killed by a vehicle, or finds his or herself in some other type of serious trouble.

Improve your training, have better control, make your life easier, avoid injuries, and ensure the safety and security of yourself and your furry best friend by choosing a Martingale collar and a standard 4-foot leash.

Sled Dog Fiasco

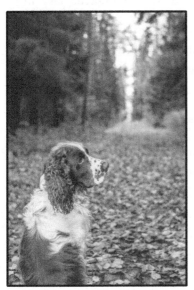

One last thought about what I call the *"Sled Dog Fiasco"*. Many people think that buying a harness is a better choice than the proper collar for their canine companion. However, the only time a harness is actually the right choice is if you have a Springer for your bicycle, or a strong sled dog that you need to put in harness, so that they can pull you.

What happens when you put most dogs in a harness is that (1) they are automatically in the wrong walking position, being head and shoulders in front of you; (2) you no longer have control of their head and cannot correct unwanted behavior; and (3) they now are in control of you and are much more powerful and potentially difficult to control, because the entire weight and strength of their body is attached to that harness.

Take Away Tip: "Harnesses are for sled dogs".

In a Nutshell

It cannot be emphasized strongly enough how important it is to properly socialize your puppy, and understand that we humans often unknowingly reward our dogs at the wrong time, which can actually cause behavioral issues later in life.

Re-visit this Chapter information and think about what other mistakes you may be inadvertently making, so that you can do your best to avoid simple mistakes we humans often are guilty of making with our dogs, that can lead to an unhappy dog that suffers from behavioral problems later in life.

Also, when training your dog, keep in mind that the type of leash and collar you choose can make a big difference.

Chapter 11: Happy English Springer Spaniel Body Language

"Money can buy a fine dog, but
only love can make him wag his tail."
— Kinky Friedman

We all know good communication is not just about the words we use. Our tone of voice, energy and our body language help to package up and deliver our meaning every day. While most people can effectively communicate their thoughts and feelings through words, we need to generally be reliant upon reading our dog's body language in order to know if they are happy, sad, nervous, afraid or aggressive.

Because our dogs don't speak our language, the only way to truly comprehend and communicate with them is for us to understand and appreciate what they are telling us through their body and vocal language.

Often, gestures or actions that we assume mean one thing are actually the dog telling us the exact opposite, and determining what that wagging tail or barking really means can sometimes be the difference between a belly rub and a bite.

How happy would you be if you could not communicate with your family at home? Would you develop behaviour issues over time? Of course you would, and the same is also true for your beloved dog.

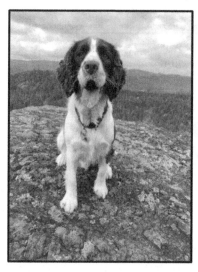

They need you to understand what they are *"telling you"* and how they feel, in order to be a happy family member. For instance, learning to properly "read" your dog's intentions can easily prevent an unwanted encounter during a visit to the local park.

Therefore, taking the time to educate yourself about basic canine body language and paying attention to your dog's body language (including their face, posture, barking and tail position) is an important prerequisite for raising a content and well-behaved dog.

This Chapter will teach you exactly that – to understand the basics of what your furry friend (and those dogs around you) are trying to *"tell"* you and how they feel, so that you can share a happy lifelong partnership together.

So, don't wait because now is a good time to start developing and honing your canine body language skills.

What's With All the Wagging and Barking?

While a well-socialized English Springer Spaniel may often happily wag their tail, it can be a mistake to automatically assume that if your dog, or someone else's dog is wagging their tail, they are happy and friendly.

What Does the Wag Mean?

When determining a dog's true intent or demeanor, it's important to take into consideration the complete dog posture, rather than just the tail, because it's entirely possible that a dog can be wagging his or her tail just before it decides to take an aggressive lunge toward you or your dog.

More important in determining the emotional state of most dogs is the height or positioning of their tail. For instance, a tail that is held parallel to your dog's back usually suggests that they are feeling relaxed, whereas if the tail is held stiffly vertical, this usually means that they may be feeling aggressive or dominant.

Also keep in mind that certain dog tails are carried differently for different reasons. Depending on which dog tail, you will have more or less visible cues. The opposite is also true of other dogs reading your dog's body language. For instance, a dog with a docked or tightly curled tail can sometimes send confusing messages to others.

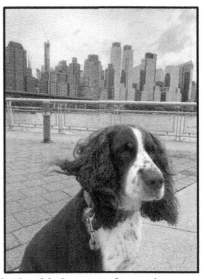

A tail held much lower can mean that your dog is feeling stressed, afraid, submissive or unwell and if the tail is tucked underneath the dog's body, this is most often a sign that the dog is feeling highly stressed, nervous, fearful or threatened by another dog, person or unfamiliar situation.

Paying attention to your dog's tail (and any dog tails around you) can help you to know when you need to step in and make some space between your dog and another, more dominant or nervous dog.

Of course, different breeds naturally carry their tails at different heights, some dogs have tightly curled tails and some dogs may not have any visible tails. You will need to take this into consideration so that you get used to their particular body language signals.

As well, the speed at which the tail is moving will give you an idea of the mental state of your dog, because the speed of the wag usually indicates how excited a dog may be.

For instance, a slow, slightly swinging wag can often mean that a dog is tentative about greeting another dog, and this is more of a questioning type of wag, whereas a fast-moving tail held high can mean that your dog is about to challenge or threaten another less dominant dog.

Also, a stalking stance, where a dog has raised hackles (hair along the back), lowers their head, crouches and slowly creeps forward with an intense stare often happens just before a serious attack. There is also a similar-looking *"play"* stance, and without practice, you may have difficulty identifying the difference between the two.

MEMORY LANE: I've been sworn at after politely letting a guardian of a larger dog, who was unaware (and didn't want to know) that their dog was stalking my smaller dog and about to do him harm, so be careful how you approach these situations.

What Does the Bark Mean?

Of course, our dogs bark for a wide variety of reasons, and every dog is different, depending upon their natural breed tendencies and how they were raised. In the case of the English Springer Spaniel, barking may occur when bored and stressed from being left alone or in excited anticipation of a walk. This section discusses some of the more common reasons why a dog might be barking.

Communication: since the very first dog, they have communicated over long distances by howling to one another and when in closer proximity, barking to warn off other dogs approaching what they consider to be their territory, or in excitement or happiness when greeting another member of the dog pack.

Now, our domesticated dogs have learned to bark for a wide variety of reasons, such as when they sense danger or are alerting us to someone approaching the home. A dog will also bark in anticipation of their favorite food, when they are afraid, frustrated, bored, excited, or to let us know they want to play. Barking is an effective way to get the attention of us humans because barking is a loud and difficult noise to ignore.

Danger: many dogs will bark to alert us to visitors or intruders, and we need to learn how to understand the difference between what our dogs perceive as danger and what is truly dangerous, or indeed how to teach our best friends the difference.

We want our dogs to tell us when there is real, imminent danger and in this case, should the danger involve an unwanted intruder, we want them to bark loudly to possibly scare this threat away.

When our dogs are barking for a reason we are not yet aware of, we need to calmly assess the situation rather than immediately becoming annoyed.

We also need to remember that the English Springer Spaniel's sense of smell, hearing and sometimes eyesight is far more acute than our own, which means that we need to give them an opportunity to tell us if they just heard, saw or sensed something that they are worried or uncertain about. The English Springer Spaniel is generally not a big barker. However, all dogs are unique, and much depends on how they were raised, so if your dog seems to be overly eager to bark at everything, you will need to take the time to teach him or her when to stop.

Rather than ignoring our dogs (or yelling at them) when they are attempting to *"tell"* us that something is bothering them, even if we ourselves understand that the noise the dog just heard is only the neighbor's kids coming home from school or a postal delivery, we need to respond appropriately.

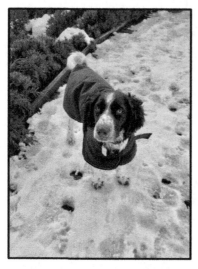

We need to calmly acknowledge our dog's concern by saying, *"OK, good dog,"* and then ask them to come to you. This way you have quietly and calmly let your dog know that the situation is nothing to be concerned about and you have asked them to move away from the target they are concerned about, which places you in control, and which will usually stop the barking.

Attention: many dogs will learn to bark to get their owner's attention, just because they are bored or want to be taken outside for an interesting walk or a trip to the local park to chase a ball.

Our canine companions are very good at manipulating us in this way, and if we fall for it, we are setting up an annoying precedent that could plague us for the remainder of our relationship.

MEMORY LANE: I shared my life with a Blue Heeler who would go berserk with loud barking every time we drove near a park or when we arrived at a park. Even so, I would never reward him for barking, because as annoying and hard on the eardrums as it was, I had to sit calmly inside the vehicle until he stopped barking. If I had let him immediately bound out of the vehicle, I would have inadvertently taught my dog that barking got him exactly what he wanted.

When a dog is barking to gain their guardian's attention, for whatever reason, before we immediately capitulate, first we need to calmly ask our dog to make eye contact with us, and do something we ask of them. After our dog has performed a calm and quiet task for us, such as sit or lie down, then we can decide to give our dog our undivided attention on our terms.

Often you will see a dog and their guardian at the local dog park playing fetch and when the human is not throwing that ball quickly enough to satisfy the dog's desire to run and fetch, the dog will be madly barking at the guardian. This is the equivalent of being sworn at in doggy language.

Don't make the mistake of allowing your puppy or dog to manipulate you in this situation, because if you do, you will soon create a bad habit that will very quickly become not just annoying to you, but also irritating to everyone else at the park.

Before throwing a ball or Frisbee for a dog that loves to chase and retrieve, it's important to always ask the dog to sit and make eye contact with you.

Often the types of canines that are overly exuberant with chasing a ball or Frisbee have usually learned this barking behavior from their humans, who allowed themselves to be literally at the beck and call of their dog, and created this noisy habit by throwing the ball every time the dog barked.

In this situation, if you allow your dog to dictate to you when you will throw the ball, they will quickly learn that barking gets them their desired result, and you have just created an annoying, rude dog who is yelling at you in doggy language to do their bidding.

In this type of ball-retrieving scenario, the dog has become ball *"obsessed"* and is no longer really paying attention to the guardian's commands, as they are solely focusing on where the ball is.

While there are many situations in which your dog may bark to convey that they've heard a noise, in all other situations where the barking is done to demand attention, a toy, other object or food, this is when you need to ask them to do something for you, and then only if you want to give them what they are asking for, do you follow through.

MEMORY LANE: I once had a client whose dog would start to loudly bark and howl every time he answered the phone. As you can imagine, this was big time annoying because nobody could hear what was being said. After a quick dog whispering session, this noisy canine companion quickly learned that this was not acceptable behavior and the problem was solved.

Bottom line, remember to stay calm when your cute puppy is demanding attention, because even negative attention can be rewarding for your dog, and can lead down a future, unwanted path where he or she will learn further habits that will not be particularly endearing for the human side of the relationship when the cute puppy has become an adult.

Boredom or Separation Anxiety: many dogs, especially those who have not been properly trained, are treated like children, are under-exercised, or that have not been allowed to understand that they have rules and boundaries, will sharply bark when left at home and are bored or are feeling the anxiety of being alone.

 Many times, we humans believe that our dog is barking when being left alone, because he or she is experiencing "separation anxiety", when in fact what the dog is really experiencing is the frustration of observing a member of the pack which they believe to be their follower (i.e. You) leaving them.

This can happen when you are not a strong enough leader for your smart English Springer Spaniel and he or she has taken over. They may then loudly verbalize their frustration and displeasure because, in the dog world, the pack <u>follower</u> (which you have allowed yourself to be) does NOT leave the pack leader (them). *I've seen this type of situation many times over, and once the human side of the relationship steps up and takes control, it quickly reverses.*

Breaking your dog of the habit of loud barking when they are left alone can be solved in different ways, with the most obvious being that you simply take your dog with you wherever you go, because after all, they are pack animals, and in order for them to be really happy and well balanced, they need the constant direction of their leader (which is supposed to be you).

Another much more lengthy and time consuming way to solve a barking problem, could involve hiring a professional to help assess why the problem has occurred in the first place and then devise an effective plan to reverse the problem that will work for each unique situation.

Fear or Pain: another reason your dog may bark is when they are very frightened or in pain and this is usually a type of bark that sounds quite different from all the others, often being a combination of a bark and a whine, or a yelping type of noise.

This is a bark that you will want to pay close attention to, so that you can quickly respond and offer the assistance that your puppy or dog may need.

Whatever reason your dog may be barking for, always remember that this is how they communicate and *"tell"* us that they want something or are concerned, afraid, nervous or unhappy about something, and as their guardians, we humans need to pay attention.

Raised Hackles: when your dog approaches with raised hackles (the hair along the dog's back), while this can be an indication that the dog may be approaching with dominant or aggressive tendencies, it also may be an indication that he or she is excited, fearful, startled, anxious or lacks confidence.

In any of these circumstances (whether it's your dog or someone else's), it's a good idea to be respectful and keep your distance until you can assess what's really going on, because even a reactive, fearful dog can quickly turn into a biting dog, and I can tell you from personal experience that being bitten by any dog really hurts.

In a Nutshell

Learning your dog's particular body language can take some time, and this Chapter will help you get started. The more you are out and about with your dog, visiting and socializing in local parks and going on walks where you will find other dogs, animals and people to observe, the more opportunity you will have to become skilled at recognizing the many subtleties of dog body language.

Paying attention to your English Springer Spaniel's verbal and body-language signals as explained above, will help you figure out what message they are trying to get across to you and this can make all the difference in preventing frustration for you both while raising a happy and well-behaved dog.

One last thought about body language and energy – check in with yourself before you walk out the door with your dog, because if you're not in the moment and have your mind on something that has nothing to do with having a successful and pleasant walk with your dog, you may be setting yourself up for trouble.

For example, if you go out the door with your dog while displaying sad, weak, fearful or confusing energy, your dog will pick up on this and become nervous or confused themselves because your energy is no longer conveying to your dog that you are their leader. This means that your energy can literally be the cause of, for instance, an uncomfortable encounter with another person walking their dog.

It's very important to keep in mind that when walking with a dog, the moment they sense that you are not completely in control, they will take this unspoken "cue" from you that being in charge has now defaulted to him or her.

You <u>never</u> want any dog to feel they must protect you from the postman, neighbor's cat or that taunting little terrier walking across the street, because if they do, you're literally out walking with a highly charged, unpredictable, live "weapon" that could decide to go off at any moment.

Most English Springer Spaniels are naturally polite and accepting of other dogs, animals and unknown people if you have put in the time to properly socialize and train them.

However, remember that this breed was originally a working gun dog that would flush prey and then retrieve it. Therefore, should you permit your dog to get seriously out of control and terrorize the neighbor's cat, for instance, you could end up with a lawsuit on your hands, and/or sky-high veterinary bills if this companion is forced into being confrontational with another animal, and that's if you're lucky.

While it would usually be a rare occurrence for the friendly English Springer Spaniel to harm someone, some of this breed can suffer from unpredictable "rage syndrome".

It's always a good idea to keep in mind that if your dog harms another dog, animal or person, or causes stress should your dog try to chase, the consequences could be far worse than a high vet bill. For instance, any dog that bites could face a death sentence or a ruling that they can never be seen in public unless they're wearing a muzzle.

Chapter 12: Training Basics for a Happy English Springer Spaniel

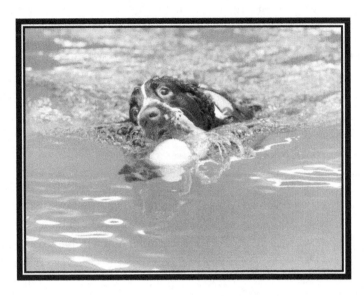

"Everyone thinks they have the best dog
in the world. None of them are wrong."
— Unknown

It's no surprise that a properly trained dog will be a much happier, safe and more secure companion that everyone enjoys being around, and that will be far less likely to develop behaviour issues later in life.

When your dog respects your leadership and there is no question that YOU are in charge, your dog can then relax and let you take the lead on training them, which is as it should be. Developing a basic training program and learning to teach your happy English Springer Spaniel commands and discipline is all part of establishing yourself as the leader and starting your dog off on the right paw.

Therefore, this Chapter will focus on training basics and tips, including hand signals, as well as simple tricks that your dog will love to learn. Take heed humans, because you will be very glad that you spent the time to learn everything contained in these pages.

All of our canine companions are amazing, natural athletes and because of this, no matter their size or breed, they need humans to lead them and daily mental and physical exercise to stay fit and healthy, so that they can be happy and well-mannered. Part of every dog's exercise routine includes learning at least three very important training basics, which are **"Come – Sit – Stay"**.

This little herding dog is a fast moving, athletic companion that can bring home the blue ribbons in several canine sports. He or she will love going for hikes, jogging, brisk walks and endless adventures with you. Most of all, these dogs will live for as much outdoor activity as possible with their guardian, and when well socialized, will also enjoy playing in a pack of other dogs.

Any type of disciplined exercise you can engage in with your dog will help to exercise both their body and their mind and will burn off pent-up daily energy reserves, so that your dog will be a happy and contented companion that is relaxed and not suffering health issues from being frustrated, under-exercised or overweight.

If you find that your dog is being a pest by chewing inappropriate items around the home or being demanding of your time, or especially unruly when visitors come to call, this is likely because their mind is not being challenged enough or their body is not being exercised often enough, vigorously enough, or long enough each day to drain out their daily pent-up energy reserves.

A healthy, adult English Springer Spaniel will thrive when being walked several times each day and mentally challenged by being engaged in other forms of disciplined canine activity, such as Agility, Flyball, Trick Training or Advanced Obedience.

This is a smart, thinking dog so use your imagination and find out what canine sports YOUR dog may enjoy learning. So long as you prove to him or her that you mean what you say through firm, fair direction and consistency, rather than too many treats, they will not feel the need to manipulate or question your authority, and will happily follow your direction.

Even at the young age of eight to ten weeks, most dogs are capable of beginning to learn anything you can teach. If you wait until they are six months old before beginning any serious training program, you could already have a stubborn problem on your hands and a wilful dog that may be unwilling to heed your commands.

 The backbone of helping to develop a well-balanced and happy English Springer Spaniel is to provide them with a routine that ensures sufficient time to satisfy their particular physical and mental exercise needs; that might include a canine sport, plus ensuring they can be with you for almost all of their time, in combination with time to play, freely run, sniff, search and explore their world every day.

What you can teach this active and agile canine companion depends entirely upon you and the time and patience you have to devote to their education, and you never want to under estimate what incredible hidden talents your dog may have.

No matter what you decide to teach, always train with firm patience, kindness, consistency and positive rewards.

It's not necessary to train with raised voices as this dog is eager to please and will quickly learn whatever you have the patience to teach.

When all training sessions are happy and fun-filled with plenty of food rewards and positive reinforcement, this will ensure that your dog is a happy, attentive student who trusts and respects you as their leader and looks forward to learning new commands, tricks and routines.

English Springer Spaniel Puppy Training Basics

First, choose a *"Discipline Sound"* that will be the same for every human family member. This will make it much easier for your puppy to learn what they can or cannot do and will be very useful when warning or redirecting your puppy before they engage in unwanted behavior.

The best types of sounds are short and sharp, so that you and your family members can quickly say them and so that the sound will immediately get the attention of your puppy, as you want to be able to easily interrupt them when they are about to make a mistake.

It doesn't really matter what the sound is, so long as it gets your dog's attention and everyone in the family is consistent. A sound that is very effective in most cases is a simple *"UH!"* sound that is said sharply and with emphasis.

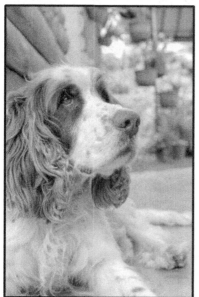

Most puppies and dogs respond immediately to this sound and if caught in the middle of doing something they are not supposed to be doing, they will quickly stop and give you their attention or back away from what they were doing.

Next, your puppy needs to learn the Three Most Important Words, which are *"Come"*, *"Sit"* and *"Stay"*. These three basic commands will ensure that your puppy remains safe in almost every circumstance.

For instance, when your puppy correctly learns the *"Come"* command, you can always quickly bring them back to you if you should see danger approaching. Also, when you teach your puppy the *"Sit"* and *"Stay"* commands, you will be further establishing your leadership role, and a puppy that understands that their human guardian is their leader will be a safe and happy follower.

Most puppies are ready to begin training at approximately 10 to 12 weeks of age (and some even earlier), so make your training sessions no more than 5 or 10 minutes (2 or 3 times a day), positive and pleasant with lots of praise and/or treats so that your puppy will be looking forward to their next session.

To help you understand the big three commands, yours truly demonstrates what the hand signals look like in the following pictures!

COME:

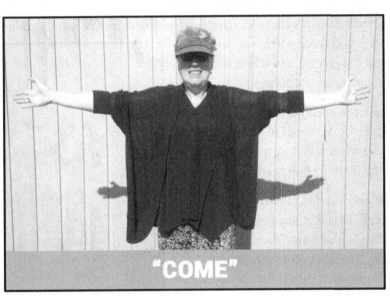

While most puppies will be capable of learning commands and tricks at a very young age, the first and most important command you need to teach your puppy is the recall, or *"Come"* command.

- ❖ Begin the *"Come"* command inside your home.

- ❖ Go into a larger room, such as your living room area.

- 🐾 Place your puppy in front of you and attach their leash or a longer line to their Martingale collar, while you back away from them a few feet.

- 🐾 Say the command *"Come"* in an excited, happy voice and hold your arms open wide.

- 🐾 If they do not immediately come to you, gently give a tug on the leash, so that they understand that they are supposed to move toward you.

- 🐾 When they come to you, happily praise them and give a treat they really enjoy.

Once your puppy can accomplish a *"Come"* command almost every time inside your home, you can then graduate them to a nearby park or quiet outside area where you will repeat the process and where there are many more distractions.

In order to keep yourself and your dog safe, he or she needs to always come to you when asked, despite whatever distractions may be nearby.

You may want to purchase an extra-long, lightweight line (25 or 50 feet), so that you are always attached to your puppy and can encourage them in the right direction should they become distracted by noises, scents and other dogs.

Try to choose a time of day when there will be fewer distractions while you are training, and remember that swiftly moving objects, dogs or other small creatures may also be a difficult distraction for this little herder to ignore.

Once your dog always comes running when called, you will no longer need to say the "Come" word, but just show them the signal, which they will be able to see from across the park

Keep in mind that even after teaching your English Springer Spaniel the *"Come"* command, their nose may take precedence over the commands you are teaching when outdoors if an interesting scent distracts them.

Always keep a young dog on leash when working in an area where they can easily run off in pursuit of an intriguing scent.

SIT:

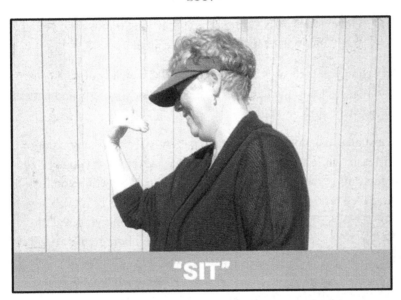

The "Sit" and *"Stay"* commands are both easy commands to teach that will help to keep your puppy safe and out of danger in almost every circumstance. Find a quiet time to teach these commands when your puppy is not overly tired.

 Ask your puppy to "Sit" and if they do not yet understand the command, show them what you mean by gently squeezing with your thumb and middle finger the area across the back that joins with their back legs.

- ❧ Do NOT just push them down into a sit, as this can cause damage to their back or joints.

- ❧ When they sit, give them a treat and praise them.

- ❧ When you say the word "Sit", at the same time show them the hand signal for this command.

- ❧ While you can use any hand signal, the universal hand signal for "Sit" is right arm (palm open facing upward) parallel to the floor, and then raising your arm while bending at the elbow toward your right shoulder.

- ❧ Once your dog is sitting reliably for you, remove the verbal "Sit" and replace it with the hand signal.

Every time you take your dog out for a walk, which is often a cause of excitement, get into the habit of asking them to sit quietly and patiently at every stage of your walk.

For instance, ask your dog to sit and patiently wait while you put on their leash, while you put on your shoes or jacket, after you approach the door, after you are on the other side of the door, while you lock the door, every time you arrive at a street intersection or crosswalk, every

time you stop during your walk to speak to a neighbor, greet a friend or admire the view, etc., and do this all in reverse when heading back home.

When you persist with the *"Sit"* training, it will soon become automatic for your dog to calmly sit every time you stop walking.

When you ask your dog to sit for you, they are learning several things all at once; that they must remain calm while paying attention to you, that you are the boss, that they must look to you for direction and that they must respect you as their leader.

Keep in mind that a sitting puppy is much easier to control than one standing at the alert, ready to bolt out the door or jump on someone. As well, because the action of sitting helps to calm the mind of an excited puppy (or dog), teaching your puppy the *"Sit"* command is a very important part of their daily interactions with your family members as well as people you may meet when out on a walk.

When you ask your puppy to *"Sit"* before you interact in any way with them, before you go out, before you feed them, etc., you are helping to quiet their mind, while teaching them to look to you for direction, and at the same time making it more difficult for them to jump, lunge or disappear out a door.

STAY:

☙ Once your puppy can reliably "Sit", say the word "Stay" (with authority in your voice) and hold your outstretched arm, palm open toward their head while backing away a few steps.

☙ If they try to follow, calmly say "No" and put them back into "Sit".

☙ Give a treat and then say again, "Stay" with the hand signal and back away a few steps.

❧ Practice these three basic "Come", "Sit", "Stay" commands everywhere you go, and use the "Sit" command as much as you can to ensure its success rate.

As your puppy gets older, and their attention span increases, you will be able to train for longer periods of time and introduce more complicated routines. This is a smart, thinking dog that can easily learn many hand signals.

Hand Signals

It's really important to use the hand signals that go along with the verbal commands during training, so that once your furry student learns both, you can remove the verbal commands in favor of just hand signals.

Hand signal training is by far the most useful and efficient training method for your dog. All too often we inundate our canine companions with a great deal of chatter and noise that they really don't understand, but because they are so willing to be part of our world, they soon learn the meaning of many words.

Contrary to what some people might think, the first language of an English Springer Spaniel (or any dog) is a combination of sensing energy and watching body language, which requires no spoken word or sound.

Therefore, when we humans take the time to teach our dog hand signals for all their basic commands, we are communicating with them at a level they instinctively understand, plus we are helping them to become a focused follower, as they must watch us in order to understand what is required of them.

Simple Tricks

When teaching your dog tricks, in order to give him or her extra incentive, find a treat that they really like and give the treat as a positive reward, which will help solidify a good performance.

Most dogs will be extra attentive during training sessions when they know that they will be rewarded with their favorite treats – especially this dog, who will usually have a healthy appetite.

If your puppy is less than six months old when you begin teaching them tricks, keep your training sessions short (no more than 5 or 10 minutes) and fun. As they become adults, you can extend your sessions, as they will be able to maintain their focus for longer periods of time.

SHAKE A PAW:

Step #1   Step #2

"Shake a Paw"

Who doesn't love a well-trained dog that knows how to shake a paw? This is one of the easiest tricks to teach your dog.

❧ Find a quiet place to practice, without noisy distractions or other pets, and stand or sit in front of your dog.

- ❧ Place them in the sitting position and have a treat in your left hand.

- ❧ Say the command "Shake" while putting your right hand behind their left or right paw and pulling the paw gently toward yourself until you are holding their paw in your hand.

- ❧ Immediately praise them and give them their favorite treat.

- ❧ Most dogs will learn the "Shake" trick quite quickly, and very soon, once you put out your hand, your dog will immediately lift their paw and put it into your hand, without your assistance or any verbal cue.

Practice every day until they are 100% reliable with this trick, and then it will be time to add another trick to their repertoire.

 __Most dogs are naturally either right or left pawed. If you know which paw your dog favors, ask them to shake this paw.__

ROLL OVER:

Step #1   Step #2   Step #3

"Roll Over" (this is circular motion)

You will find that just as your dog is naturally either right or left pawed, they will also naturally want to roll either to the right or the left side. Take advantage of this by asking your dog to roll to the side they naturally prefer.

- Sit with your dog on the floor and put them in a lie down position.

- Hold a treat in your hand and place it close to their nose without allowing them to grab it.

- While they are in the lying position, move the treat to the right or left side of their head (the nose will follow the treat), so that they have to roll over to get to it.

- You will very quickly see which side they want to naturally roll to, and once you see this, move the treat to this side.

- When they roll over to this side, immediately give them the treat and praise them.

- You can say the verbal cue "Over" while you demonstrate the hand signal motion (moving your right hand in a circular motion) or moving the treat from one side of their head to the other with a half circle motion.

SIT PRETTY:

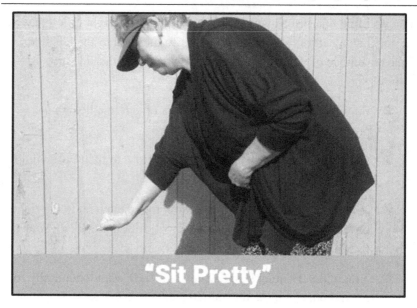

"Sit Pretty"

While this trick is a little more complicated, and most dogs pick up on it very quickly, remember that every dog is different so always exercise patience.

- Find a quiet space with few distractions and sit or stand in front of your dog and ask them to "Sit".

- Have a treat nearby (on a countertop or table) and when they sit, use both of your hands to lift up their front paws into the sitting pretty position, while saying the command "Sit Pretty".

- Help them balance in this position, while you praise them and give them the treat.

- Once your dog can perform the balancing part of the trick quite easily without your help, sit or stand in front of your dog while asking them to "Sit Pretty".

- Holding the treat above their head at the level of their nose would be when they sit pretty.

- If they attempt to stand on their back legs to get the treat, you may be holding the treat too high, which will encourage them to stand on their back legs to reach it. Go back to the first step and put them back into the "Sit" position and again lift their paws while their backside remains on the floor.

❧ After they learn the trick on verbal command, try saying the verbal cue while demonstrating the hand signal: holding your straight arm, fully extended, over your dog's head with a closed fist (pictured).

❧ Make this a fun and entertaining time for both of you and practice a few times every day until they can "Sit Pretty" on hand signal command every time you ask.

A smart young puppy should be able to easily learn these basic tricks before they are six months old and when you are patient and make your training sessions short and fun for your dog, they will be eager to learn so much more.

Crate Training

The best method for housetraining your dog is called crate training. Basically, you give your puppy many opportunities to do his or her business outside, so they are not tempted to do it inside. During times when you cannot keep a constant watch on your puppy (such as when you're making dinner or sleeping), you put him or her in their crate as this will help to prevent hidden accidents elsewhere in your house. As long as you use the crate for this purpose and you help your puppy form a positive association with the crate, he or she will not mind being in it. Just do not use it as a form of punishment!

So, how exactly do you go about house training your puppy? Here's a step-by-step guide:

1. Choose a certain part of your yard where you want your dog to go.

2. Take your puppy outside every hour or so -- directly to the chosen spot every time.

3. When you take your puppy out, say "Go pee" as soon as you set him or her down in that area.

4. Wait for your puppy to do his business – and the moment they do, immediately praise them in an excited voice and give a small treat as a reward.

5. If your puppy does not have to go, take them back inside instead of letting him wander around.

6. When you're at home, keep a close eye on your puppy and confine them to whatever room you are in.

7. Watch your dog for signs that he or she has to go and take them outside immediately if they start to sniff the ground, walk in circles, or squat.

8. During times when you cannot physically watch your puppy, put him or her in their crate to reduce the risk of an accident – do not keep any food or water in the crate with them.

9. Let your puppy go outside to relieve his or herself immediately before putting them in the crate and also immediately after releasing them. You should also take your puppy outside shortly after a meal or when they wake up from a nap.

10. Take away your puppy's food and water about an hour before bedtime until they are able to go the whole night without an accident.

When you first bring your puppy home, you shouldn't expect him or her to be able to hold their bladder or bowels for more than an hour or two. Even so, you should start crate training right away so they learn good habits from an early age. As they get older, they will be able to wait longer before needing a bathroom break – about one hour for each month of age.

Adult Training

The English Springer Spaniel is a dog that will thrive so long as they are getting to spend fun time and activities close to their human. Therefore, in order to ensure a happy and healthy dog that will not develop behaviour issues out of boredom or laziness, make sure that you get your dog involved in interesting activities, such as Advanced Obedience, Trick Training, Agility, Flyball or perhaps Dock Diving.

When your dog is a full-grown adult (approximately two years of age), you will definitely want to begin more complicated or advanced training sessions.

When you have the desire and patience, you may be surprised at how many commands, tricks, routines or canine sports you can teach a happy, willing English Springer Spaniel who trusts and respects their human guardian.

For instance, you may wish to teach your adult dog more advanced tricks, such as opposite sided paw shakes or rollovers, which are more difficult than you might expect and which this athletic dog is definitely capable of learning.

If you and your dog are really enjoying learning new tricks or routines together, consider teaching them a series of hand signals, such as *"Commando crawl"*, *"Speak"* or *"Jump through the human hoop"*, or perhaps get them certified as a therapy dog so they can brighten the days of those who must spend time in hospitals and care facilities.

Teaching your dog tricks and routines builds trust and respect, is fun for both of you, and a healthy way to exercise both your dog's mind and body, which will result in a happy, contented and well-behaved companion.

Over-Exercising

Be especially careful about over-exercising your fur friend when it's warm out and when they are really young (as their muscles and bones are not yet fully developed), because like humans, dogs can also collapse from heat stroke.

Playtime

Every dog needs some down time or regular playtime each day, and while every dog will be different with respect to what types of games they may enjoy, most will really love any game involving retrieving a ball or soft toy.

The super smart English Springer Spaniel may also be a very excited participant in a fun game of *"Search"*, where you ask your dog to *"Sit/Stay"* while you hide a favorite treat that they then have to use their nose to find.

To begin teaching the "Search" game, first time ask your dog to sit/stay while you slowly back away and place a treat where they can actually still see it. Return to where they are in their sit/stay and say, "OK! Search!" and point to where you just placed the treat. Each time you play this game, you can place the treat farther and farther away and completely out of their sight before you release them to "Search!"

After a disciplined walk with your dog, they will also enjoy being given the opportunity for some off-leash freedom to really stretch out by running free to play and socialize with other similar-sized dogs at the local dog park.

In a Nutshell

Taking the time to teach your dog basic rules and boundaries and always firmly enforce them, plus simple or complex tricks and interesting tasks to keep their mind engaged, will keep them both mentally and physically healthy and happy and you will raise a well-behaved dog that is a joy to be around.

While the English Springer Spaniel can appear to have a stubborn streak or be strong-willed, this is usually because he or she is very smart and easily bored. If you are consistently confident and firm, he or she will be an eager to please, willing to learn dog with a loyal, loving personality.

In order to ensure a healthy, happy and contented dog that is not overweight and will not develop behavior issues out of boredom or neglect, you must take the time to involve them in daily moderate to high physical and mental exercise that can include different activities, such as interesting canine sports where they get to develop their unique skills.

Chapter 13: What If You Slip Up?

"Dogs got personality.
Personality goes a long way."
— Quentin Tarantino

All the information, suggestions, tips and advice given in this book is the result of more than 40 years experience helping humans positively and effectively interact with the canine world.

If you take all that is written on these pages to heart, and regularly and consistently apply them, your English Springer will grow up to be a happy family member that will not have to suffer from any behavioral issues.

However, if your lifestyle drastically changes, you forget to exercise your dog, keep on top of basic or advanced training, or you slip up for any number of reasons, problems may inevitably occur.

For instance, you may end up becoming too busy or distracted with your human life to provide your canine companion with what he or she needs on a daily basis to be a happy and fulfilled member of your family.

Realistically, there may be any number of other reasons why you may not consistently apply the information given here, and the following is an outline of just a few of the more common behavioral issues that could occur, with some tips that may help you get back on track.

When reading the following pages, please keep in mind that a specific behavioral problem is usually the result of many different possibilities or circumstances that have taken place between the human individual or family and the particular dog.

This means that properly addressing a specific unwanted behavior often needs the assistance of a professional with a personal approach, who can ask the right questions to determine how the unwanted behavior occurred, because it's often not what you may have initially thought.

Therefore, to generically outline possible ways to reverse an unwanted behavior will be a guessing game, because without knowing the circumstances of the guardian and their family, and understanding the situation that triggered the unwanted behavior, I can only make my best guess based on previous experience with similar problems.

As an example, there might be many reasons why the dog in question is chewing the tassels on your Persian rug. For instance, this could be because they:

- are hungry
- are teething
- have a taste for wool
- think the tassels are a toy

- are a super high energy dog

- are left alone and are bored

- haven't been given appropriate toys to chew

- have not been taught rules and what is appropriate

- need a guardian with stronger leadership energy

- are bored and under-exercised

- are over-stimulated

As you can see, it's possible for almost endless scenarios and reasons why a dog may develop a particular behavioral issue.

Therefore, please understand that without close observation and much more information explaining a particular situation, the following few common behavioral problems and the suggestions for alleviating them, will be my best guess.

Chewing Inappropriate Items
[Re-visit *"Distraction and Replacement"* in Chapter 10]

If your puppy or dog is chewing the carpet, your fingers, the legs of the coffee table, your shoes, or any other inappropriate item(s) that are not dog toys, rather than getting upset with your dog, you need to train yourself to be much more vigilant, and then distract and replace.

First make sure that all the chewing is not just because the puppy is teething. Have compassion because teething is painful for the puppy and they must chew to help alleviate the pain while those adult teeth are growing in.

Always make sure your puppy has plenty of chew toys and to help with the teething pain, give your puppy an old T-towel soaked in water, tied in knots and frozen in the freezer as a chew toy.

When your dog is a little older, already has pushed through their adult set of teeth and has decided, for instance, that the legs on your coffee table are good chew toys, it is possible that you:

- 🐾 are not paying attention and taking the time to make sure your dog receives enough vigorous daily exercise, and/or,

- 🐾 are not teaching your dog what is, and what is not, appropriate for chewing by saying a firm and convincing "No", replacing the table leg with a toy they are allowed to chew, and praising them when they've got the right thing between their teeth.

Being Fearful of Loud Noises
[Re-visit *"Fear of Loud Noises"* in Chapter 10]

If you have raised a dog that has a fear of loud, popping noises, perhaps you haven't taken the time to read this information and apply the suggestions outlined, so read it now and practice until your dog loses or at least diminishes their fear.

Excessive Excitement When Friends Visit
[Re-visit *"Chapter 3: Overview of the Happy English Springer Spaniel"* and *"Chapter 12: Training Basics for a Happy English Springer Spaniel"*]

Make sure that you begin to teach an excitable young dog to be a calm follower as soon as you bring him or her home.

Always ignore an excited dog and do <u>not</u> touch them until they are calm and relaxed, otherwise you will inadvertently teach them that it is acceptable behavior for them to be excited every time they see a human.

If they are overly excited when friends come to visit, stand between your dog and your friends, and create some space by pointing away and firmly telling your dog, "*GO*", and also ask your friends to ignore him or her.

Also, if you've been properly training your puppy or dog, you will have taught them to *"Sit"* on command, and a sitting dog is much more relaxed and easier to control.

Acting Aggressively on a Walk
[Re-visit *"Chapter 12: Training Basics for a Happy English Springer Spaniel"*]

Make sure that your dog is walking at your side without pulling on the leash when you are out for a walk.

When you train your dog to walk beside you, this *"tells"* them that YOU are their leader and in charge of every situation, which means they will be much less likely to act out or attempt to "protect" you from outside stimuli. If they DO try, immediately give a sharp tug on that Martingale collar along with a strong "*NO!*" to remind them who is the boss.

Pulling When on Leash
[Re-visit *"The Martingale Collar"* in Chapter 10]

If your dog is pulling on leash, chances are high that he or she is not wearing the proper training collar and you have not taken the time to teach them to quietly walk at your side.

Buy your dog a Martingale collar, properly adjust it, and then the next time they try to pull ahead of you, give a sharp snap to this collar (toward yourself) and firmly say the word "*Heel*".

Repeating this process until your dog understands can take a few minutes or even several days, as each dog is different – be consistent and persistent until your dog gets it.

Also, turning circles or figure eights and changing directions suddenly when on a leash walk will quickly help to teach your dog their proper walking position, because if they are ahead of you they are going to be stepped on or walked into.

Stealing Food or Raiding the Garbage Can

[Re-visit *"Ideal Living Conditions for a Happy English Springer Spaniel"* in Chapter 6]

Make sure you absolutely understand that the English Springer Spaniel may be a highly food motivated breed, and an athletic dog will have no difficulty jumping up on counter tops. If given the opportunity and the food is enticing enough, any dog will steal food. This means that in order to avoid this possibility, you must be a vigilant guardian and make sure that you never leave any food they should not eat unattended or where they can reach it.

Not Obeying Commands

[Re-visit *"Chapter 12: Training Basics for a Happy English Springer Spaniel"*]

A well-trained English Springer Spaniel is one that obeys the basic *"Come/Sit/Stay"* commands. If your dog is not obeying your commands, you have not taken the time to properly train them, or you are too weak a leader, with the result being that he or she will take a stubborn attitude, they will ignore you and they will not respect you as their leader.

Get to work right away, step up your energy to ensure you are a strong enough leader, and train your dog so that everyone will be happy.

 We all have our off days, so don't get down on yourself if you occasionally slip up and are not being as vigilant, strong

and confident a leader as you need to be with this dog's basic and/or advanced training and daily maintaining of rules and boundaries.

In a Nutshell

We humans will always have days when we are not as vigilant as we need to be, which means that we will inevitably "slip up" sometimes when raising our fur friends.

What you need to remember is that it's not the end of the world, because there is always a solution, and often simply re-reading the relevant chapters in this book can quickly and easily get you back on track to raising a happy and well-behaved English Springer Spaniel that is a pleasure to be around.

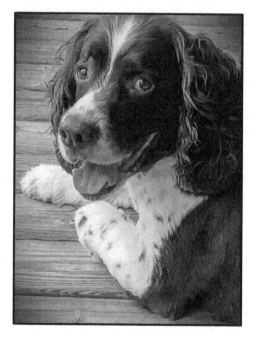

Also, know that the familiar expression, "You can't teach an old dog new tricks," is totally false. It doesn't matter what age a particular dog may be, because with patience and the right energy and knowledge, you absolutely CAN teach a dog of any age new tricks. It's us humans that have difficulties learning new tricks.

Chapter 14: Surprise Bonus Chapter

*"Dogs have a way of finding the people
who need them, and filling an emptiness
we didn't ever know we had."*
— Thom Jones

If you thought that you had reached the end of this book, well surprise, not quite yet, as I'd like to leave you with some canine wisdom and a short, funny, true story.

Happy English Springer Spaniel Question and Answer (Q&A) section

The following Question and Answer (Q&A) section is written from the dog's perspective, and although you may find it amusing, there are also valuable human lessons to be learned, if anyone is paying attention.

First, let me set the scene for the following situations:

This is a young, busy family, consisting of Mom and Dad, who work at home, one 12-year-old girl, and one 14-year-old boy, who share their lives with a neutered, 2-year-old dog named Harvey. They all live together in a large house with a medium-sized, fenced yard out the back.

The following questions, asked by various members of the family, are directed to the dog, and answered by the dog, as if the dog could talk like their humans.

Each question the dog answers is followed by a short synopsis of the "lesson" we humans can learn from these various interactions.

Mom: **"Oh No! Why did you pee on the floor?"**

Harvey: *"I'm sorry, I didn't mean to, but you forgot to let me out before everyone left for that baseball game, and I just couldn't hold it any longer."*

Lesson: Humans often lead very busy and distracted lives, and in order to ensure their dog remains happy, they still need to always pay attention and put their canine friend's habits and needs ahead of their own.

Girl: **"Yuckeeee! Harvey, why do you smell like dog poo?"**

Harvey: *"I was chasing a squirrel in the back yard, as much as I tried to tiptoe through those piles of doggy doo that the boy hadn't picked up yet in the back yard, I guess I accidentally stepped in one."*

Lesson: Humans with convenient back yard doggy bathrooms often forget to be vigilant about picking up the yard. This is not only a smelly bad habit that busy (or lazy) guardians are guilty of, it's also a considerable health hazard that attracts rats.

Boy: **"What's wrong, Harvey? You like to fetch — go get that ball!"**

Harvey: *"Yes, I like to fetch, but it's hot out here, I'm getting exhausted and if I don't get water soon, I may pass out."*

Lesson: Sometimes we humans sharing our lives with dogs that have great stamina tend to forget that the temperature of the day, that doesn't seem extreme to us, can quickly be too much for a dog that is running back and forth fetching a ball while we're standing still. We also forget that many dogs, despite their discomfort, like to please their humans and may continue to fetch that ball even though they may be about to collapse from heat exhaustion and are dying of thirst.

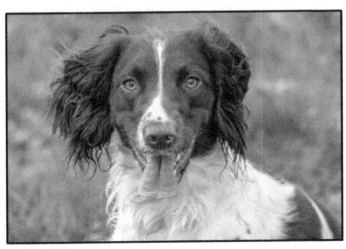

Dad: **"What happened in here, Harvey! You've made a huge mess of all these boxes I had neatly stacked in the carport! What's wrong with you?"**

Harvey: *"I saw a squirrel in here eating through the boxes and I was just trying to protect the home. I finally got rid of him, and he won't be coming back. Sorry I knocked over the boxes."*

Lesson: Often we tend to quickly blame our canine friends when a mess is created for which there seems to be no explanation. We need to first think beyond simply blaming the dog for unexplained disarray, as there is often a good explanation that, in most cases, exonerates your canine companion.

Mom: **"Harvey! What have you done? I left a plate of cheese and crackers on the coffee table for our guests. Did you eat them?"**

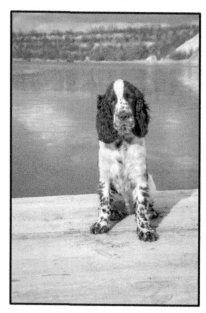

Harvey: *"I smelled them when I was passing through the kitchen and couldn't resist. I love cheese and the crackers were OK too, but now I think I might have to throw up."*

Lesson: Many of our canine companions (such as the English Springer Spaniel) don't know when to stop when it comes to filling their stomach. Therefore, if you have one of these dogs with an endless appetite for anything remotely resembling food, you need to be vigilant about never leaving human food, garbage or anything edible where they can reach it.

Boy: **"You bad, bad dog, Harvey! You've chewed the laces off my expensive tennis shoes."**

Harvey: *"But they smell just the same as those old shoes you gave me to play with, and now you're mad at me? Someone's confused."*

Lesson: Think about what you allow your canine friend to play with, because giving them old discarded shoes, socks or other articles of clothing, etc., to play with causes confusion in the canine mind when you get mad if they decide to chew your new shoes.

Girl: **"You're covering my bed in mud Harvey! Get out!"**

Harvey: *"But I like being next to you, and you let me sleep on your bed when I was a puppy, so please let me up."*

Lesson: If you'd rather not share your bed with a dog that could have just walked through a muddy puddle, don't make the mistake of allowing them to sleep with you when they're a cute and much smaller cuddly puppy. If you do, it's unfair to blame your canine companion for wanting to continue this habit that you literally taught them.

Dad: **"Are you kidding me, Harvey? Where's the steaks I left on the picnic table!"**

Harvey: *"There were circling crows and I tried to chase them away, but they smelled so good that I couldn't resist. I'm sorry – I ate them while you were getting a beer. They were so delicious - got any more?"*

Lesson: Dogs are carnivorous and no matter their size, whether a tiny Chihuahua, a large Mastiff, or a hungry English Springer Spaniel, if given the opportunity, their desire to eat meat is a strong instinct they cannot ignore. If you leave meat unattended, and your dog eats it, too bad stupid human - don't blame your canine companion.

Moral of the Q&A section

Always DO pay attention to what your dog is trying to tell you, because (in addition to the above), there are so many other lessons we humans can learn from our beloved canine companions. Watching out and learning these lessons and appropriately acting upon them, will help you to raise a Happy English Springer Spaniel that will never have to experience unwanted behaviors.

There are so many lessons we humans can learn from our beloved canine companions IF we are paying attention.

Happy English Springer Spaniel True Story

Before we close this Chapter, I hope you will enjoy the following true short story:

Ozzy's New Tiles

I was dog-sitting Ozzy, the English Springer Spaniel, for clients of mine who had just recently installed a new tile entranceway in their home where previously there had been carpet tiles. The owners warned me that they were having a *"little problem"* getting Ozzy used to the new, shiny and quite slippery tiles and I told them not to worry about it, as I presumed this was a minor issue.

However, I soon found out that the joke was on me, because once I had delivered Ozzy's owners to the airport and I returned to the home with Ozzy on leash at my side and I opened the front door, I was brought to a sudden abrupt halt when Ozzy refused to enter the house.

Ozzy stopped so suddenly that all the groceries I was carrying became airborne and ended up strewn across the floor while it felt like I had suddenly become attached to a wriggling fire hydrant. OK, so much for the *"little"* problem Ozzy was having with the new flooring because he flatly refused to put even one paw on those shiny new tiles.

Thank goodness it was a pleasant summer day because now was the time to start working out Ozzy's fear of shiny surfaces and this meant keeping the front door open.

I tied Ozzy's leash to the railing near the door, rescued my groceries from the tiled floor, found some of Ozzy's favorite treats, and returned to untie Ozzy while I showed him I had something he wanted. He was immediately interested in the treats and started to follow me into the house only to abruptly stop at the door.

I went inside a couple of feet and sat down with his treats on the tiled surface, holding my hand out to offer him one. He stretched as far as he could without stepping on the tiles trying to get to the treats he really wanted, while I kept calmly encouraging him to move forward.

Finally, after several failed attempts to get him to put a paw on the dreaded tile surface, he completely flattened himself onto his belly and used his legs like a frog to *"swim"* his way across the tiles to get the treats I was offering.

This was definitely one of the funniest things I had ever seen a dog do, but I had to be careful not to laugh because he needed me to be his strong and confident leader, so I stifled my laughter and praised him for being so brave.

So now here was Ozzy flat on his belly in the middle of the shiny tile surface with his beloved carpeting about ten slippery tiles away. I stood up and moved farther into the house onto the carpeted area, still encouraging him to come and get his favorite treats.

He stared at me with those pleading eyes that seemed to say *"help me out of this predicament"*, and all I could do was talk softly and confidently to him, pretending everything was just fine as I asked him to come and get his treats.

After a couple of minutes, Ozzy decided that the only way to get what he wanted was to *"swim"* a little farther and he flailed with his front paws and kicked with his back feet like a frog until he made his way onto the carpet, where he immediately bounded into life.

Stifling my laughter, I immediately praised and petted him, gave him several of his favorite treats, and all was now right in Ozzy's world, until it came time to go out for a lunchtime walk around the block.

I hitched up Ozzy's leash to his Martingale collar and started to walk toward the front door, which involved crossing over the tiled entranceway, hoping he would forget about his fear, but as soon as we reached the edge of the carpet, he immediately put the brakes on.

I stopped with him, keeping some forward tension on his leash, as I offered him a treat if he would just take one step onto the tiles. Instead, he immediately dropped onto his belly again, like a penguin about to slide down a snow bank, and started pushing himself across the tiles to get to the treat I was offering.

Such a sight he was and so determined to get his treat without having to walk – you had to give him credit for his amazing ingenuity.

When he got to my outstretched hand and gobbled down his treat, I gently picked him up and placed his feet onto the dreaded tiles and again encouraged him to walk toward me. This time, although he remained crouched low, he gingerly attempted his first step, and then another and another until you could actually see a light bulb go off in his doggy brain when he realized that the smooth surface of the tiles was indeed safe to walk on.

I happily praised him for his bravery and gave him another treat, and then a few more times in and out the door and although he would slightly hesitate when stepping onto the tiles, and stoop down to sniff them, within three days of practicing our little routine, the dreaded slippery tile flooring was no longer a problem for this smart Springer Spaniel.

When his owners returned from their holiday, you can imagine how happy they were to know that they no longer had to carry Ozzy across their entranceway.

Lesson to learn: **No matter the age of your dog, and how much you may have socialized them, when you change something in their world, they can become nervous, scared and traumatized. The only way to work through this is with much patience and understanding, coupled with persistent calm energy, and of course, favorite treats.**

Chapter 15: Conclusion and Reviews

"Once you have a wonderful dog,
a life without one is a life diminished."
— Dean Koontz

This book is written to help anyone thinking of sharing their life with the versatile, smart and energetic English Springer Spaniel, to first understand whether or not they truly have the time, energy and lifestyle that would be compatible with raising a healthy and happy dog.

Once it's been decided that this versatile canine is the right breed to share your life with, the purpose of this book is to help you understand how to properly care for an English Springer Spaniel.

This will include socializing, training and providing this dog with adequate physical and mental daily exercise, the best food, regular clipping and a safe environment, so that this dog can live the longest and most contented life possible.

There are already plenty of books written, and many different trainers and opinions concerning how to correct a dog that may be suffering from any number of behavioral issues.

However, to my knowledge, there are no breed-specific books that take the time to outline how most issues that could have been avoided, have instead been inadvertently created by the dog's human guardian. Therefore, this breed-specific book stands out from all other current publications, because it:

- highlights that almost all problems, both mentally and physically, are a direct result of ignorance, lack of research, unwillingness or inability on the part of the human guardian to give their chosen dog what he or she truly needs.

- describes in detail what the human guardian needs to understand and commit to doing on a daily basis in order to match the English Springer Spaniel's needs, so that they can raise a happy, healthy and well-behaved dog that never has to experience behavioral issues.

There is much knowledge for this breed contained within the pages of this book that has been gained over some 40 years working with dogs. This information will help anyone serious about raising a *HAPPY* English Springer Spaniel, so that they can easily implement all the practical tips of this book without having to hire a professional to help them correct any sort of future behavioral problems.

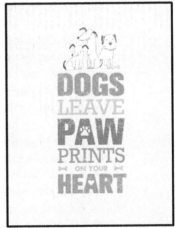

In a nutshell, this book contains all you need to raise a Happy English Springer Spaniel that will never have to experience unwanted behaviors or end up behind bars at the local SPCA.

What Past Clients Have to Say

The following are a few happy reviews from some of my past dog whispering clients, who did the work required to turn their chosen fur friend into a happy and well-behaved companion. I have taught these clients how to apply some of the tips and techniques described in this book (such as how to establish yourself as the pack leader) and they easily managed to get back on track to raising a happy and well-behaved companion.

Thus, rather than taking my word for the effectiveness of the methods contained in this book, perhaps you would prefer to take my clients' word!!

> *"Thank you for your report and teaching me to be a pack leader ... this has worked remarkably as Drew and Sammy have responded well beyond my expectations... Drew is very calm and relaxed and our walks are now very enjoyable...*
>
> *I want you to know that I really appreciate your help... Results have been spectacular and both dogs have evolved into superheroes and have accepted me as their pack leader and respond positively..."*
> ~ Klaus, Drew, Sammy & Max the Cat
>
> *"I just wanted to thank you again for our lesson today. You really are amazing with dogs. Tim and I learned so much from you, it's really neat to see the difference it makes in the dogs when you take control..."*
> ~ Morgan, Tim, Grizzly, Bella & Bear
>
> *"I was at the point I was ready to give Jake away because I was so concerned about how he reacted every time someone came to the door. It was really embarrassing! Honestly, within three hours of Asia being here, Jake was a different dog. We learned how to become the pack leader and control him..."*
> ~ Sharon, Mike & Jake
>
> *"My partner and I and our dog Rollo recently moved to Victoria from up north. Rollo, unused to city life and walking on a leash, was nervous and reactive around other dogs. Asia showed us how we need to behave so he could relax. After just one session the difference was very impressive – walks have become relaxing and enjoyable again – for all of us..."*
> ~ Tim, Mary & Rollo
>
> *"Thank you for helping me become the guardian that Ida needs. She was a good dog to start with, now she is an incredible dog.*

She walks well on lead, stays in my unfenced yard, and comes when called. I am often complimented on what a well-behaved dog I have. Thanks for making it all happen..."
~ Kristiane & Ida

Published by Worldwide Information Publishing 2020